Care*fair*

Paul Kershaw

Care*fair*
Rethinking the Responsibilities
and Rights of Citizenship

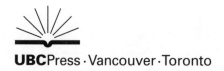

UBCPress · Vancouver · Toronto

15 14 13 12 11 10 09 08 07 06 05   5 4 3 2 1

Printed in Canada on acid-free paper

Library and Archives Canada Cataloguing in Publication

Kershaw, Paul W. (Paul William), 1974-
  Carefair : rethinking the responsibilities and rights of citizenship / Paul Kershaw.

Includes bibliographical references and index.
ISBN 0-7748-1160-9 (bound); ISBN 0-7748-1161-7 (pbk.)

  1. Work and family – Canada. 2. Canada – Social policy. 3. Caregivers – Canada.
4. Child care – Canada. 5. Sex role – Canada. 6. Citizenship – Social aspects. 7.
Feminist ethics. I. Title.

HV108.K47 2005   306.85′0971   C2005-901188-2

Canadä

UBC Press gratefully acknowledges the financial support for our publishing program of the Government of Canada through the Book Publishing Industry Development Program (BPIDP), and of the Canada Council for the Arts, and the British Columbia Arts Council.

This book has been published with the help of a grant from the Canadian Federation for the Humanities and Social Sciences, through the Aid to Scholarly Publications Programme, using funds provided by the Social Sciences and Humanities Research Council of Canada, and with the help of the K.D. Srivastava Fund.

Printed and bound in Canada by Friesens
Set in Stone by Artegraphica Design Co. Ltd.
Copy editor: Audrey McClellan
Proofreader: Dallas Harrison
Indexer: Noeline Bridge

UBC Press
The University of British Columbia
2029 West Mall
Vancouver, BC V6T 1Z2
604-822-5959 / Fax: 604-822-6083
www.ubcpress.ca

From Andrea and Paul to Ryan Alexander Lloyd-Doust,
the first child born to our dear friends, Simone and Micheal ...

in full confidence that you will witness and profit from the care*fair* ideal because your parents foreshadow the social change this manuscript prescribes. Their daily care for you is not just a private blessing, but also a public virtue that subverts persistent patriarchal norms and illuminates alternative gender patterns for fellow citizens. Let this be the first of many lessons that the personal is political! The book is also testament to all the care to which you are entitled from Andrea and me in our dual role as extended family and citizens. But since rights entail responsibilities, let the book further stimulate you to consider what we and others can ultimately expect from you as you mature, grapple with masculine norms, and inherit a social order that we hope will some day integrate care, gender equality, and work-family balance as constitutive responsibilities and rights of Canadian citizenship.

Contents

Acknowledgments

Since no single-authored book is a solo project, I am indebted to a web of relations and institutional supports in and beyond academia that have facilitated my research in recent years. Emily Andrew, senior editor at UBC Press, exemplifies all that one could hope for from an editor when embarking on a first book, including experience, skill, grace, patience, and timely correspondence. Audrey McClellan performed yeoman's service editing the manuscript, and Darcy Cullen ensured that it travelled through the publication process without a hitch.

The Social Sciences and Humanities Research Council (SSHRC) financially supported Care*fair* from its genesis onward. A grant from the Council's Postdoctoral Fellowship competition subsidized the time I required to research and write the manuscript. The Equality, Security and Community Project and the Consortium for Health, Intervention, Learning and Development, both funded through the SSHRC Major Collaborative Initiatives, cultivated an invigorating pan-Canadian scholarly community in which I could develop and present some of the core themes around which the book is organized. Funding from the Council's Aid to Scholarly Publications Programme saw the project to its completion by helping to finance publication costs. The manuscript's publication is one example of the SSHRC's success at supporting emerging interdisciplinary scholars.

The book also benefited enormously from the stimulating intellectual home that the Human Early Learning Partnership (HELP) made available through its postdoctoral program. Living up to its acronym, the partnership helped to nurture my scholarship during the hectic period of manuscript writing and revision. HELP is funded by a grant from the British Columbia Ministry of Children and Family Development. Special thanks to HELP's associate director, Hillel Goelman, and its director, Clyde Hertzman, for their generous and ongoing mentoring.

Barbara Arneil, Claire Young, Jon Kesselman, and Kathy Teghtsoonian provided insightful, cogent, and frank feedback about sections in early drafts of the manuscript. They graciously demonstrated patience, flexibility, and expertise supporting a young colleague who did not (want to?) fit into one set of disciplinary boundaries. David Wu proved to be a remarkably detailed and conscientious research assistant whose work was tremendously valuable for completing the bibliography and citations. Despite this support, the standard proviso stands: any errors in the book are mine alone.

As Care*fair* is integrated into course syllabi, it is fitting to acknowledge three scholars who took the time to develop superb courses that continue to shape the way I think about many of the themes that are examined in this book: David Kahane in his course "Justice and Cultural Diversity in Contemporary Canadian Political Theory"; Susan Dwyer in her course "Feminist Epistemology"; and Susan Boyd in her course at UBC "Feminist Legal Theory: Key Themes and Current Debates." While "publish or perish" signals the path to academic success, each of these professors also sets a tremendously high teaching standard that I wish to emulate as I continue my own career in the classroom.

Beyond the world of academia, I am beholden to a network of family and friends too numerous to name who helped me withstand the endurance test that is a book. Some relationships stand out, including the stalwart support of my parents Sue, Don, Ann, John, and Ruth, and my in-laws, Chris and Gloria. Although the arguments in this book target the need to revise male care practices, I would be remiss not to single out the devotion of my mother, whose care has been a constant that all sons and daughters should have the good fortune to benefit from.

In a society where blood relations are fragile, I am proud to count in my extended family some cherished friends who contributed implicitly to the writing process. Simone and Mike never failed to show genuine interest in my manuscript and gave me a chance to examine multiple ideas over many a relaxing drink. They also represent an inspiring spousal, and now parental, relationship that influenced my thinking about gender equality and societal time rhythms. Brian is the first friend I learned to trust unconditionally, and his frequent visits, with Christine, remain foundational for revealing the value of work-life balance.

Finally, I know not the words (which will not surprise her) to describe the debt I owe my partner Andrea. I marvel at her strength of will, which fuels my own, as well as the subtlety of her intellect, which illuminates the nuances of scholarly texts and, more importantly, my lived experience. No other person's writing or thinking has factored more prominently in shaping my own, in part because she helped me understand that "it's in the details." May I live up to the masculine care ideals set forth in this book as we continue to interweave our lives at our new Homecoming Farm.

1
Lamenting the Lazy Lavatory Syndrome: Political Theory, Policy, and Civic Virtue

The lazy lavatory syndrome refers to a peculiar, but apparently not uncommon, ailment in the office building in which I work at the University of British Columbia, Canada. Throughout the building, the washroom entrances, cubicle doors, and bathroom mirrors are adorned with signs asking all visitors to "Please Flush after Every Use." A female colleague has confirmed that the signage is not a decorative feature of the men's rooms only.

Not surprisingly, the signs attract graffiti. Some of this includes intelligent political debate concerning the sustainability of the university's human waste management system in the midst of water shortages that have afflicted British Columbia during recent summer droughts. But despite the acumen that informs the bathroom break exchange, no one denounces what I believe is the most jarring political reality signalled by the signs: some of the most privileged, learned citizens in our society are so dismissive of the obligations one must fulfill to sustain the communities that make privilege possible that they require regular reminders to take responsibility for disposing of their own waste rather than free riding off the flushing of fellow citizens.

The (momentary?) absence of civility that characterizes the lazy lavatory syndrome is symbolic of the alleged decline of civic-spiritedness with which much normative political discourse has engaged over the past two decades. Kymlicka and Norman (1994, 352; 2000, 5; 2003) document this reorientation in their series of review articles analyzing the "explosion of interest in the concept of citizenship" that emerged in the 1990s. In contrast to scholarship about Rawlsian theories of justice and the resulting focus on basic social institutions that dominated Anglo-American political philosophy into the late 1980s, the analytic shift toward citizenship signalled renewed recognition among theorists that citizenry qualities, attitudes, and Tocquevilleian "habits of the heart" are also integral to the health and stability of modern democracies. Attention to civic virtues and the social duties they imply emerged across political camps, including among "third way" scholars toward the left of centre, neoliberals and social conservatives on the right, as well as new communitarians and feminists for whom the left/right divide offers a less than satisfactory categorical framework. Among the many virtues identified, theorists accorded prominent interest to citizens' willingness to accept responsibility for personal choices that affect the broader community and environment, particularly with respect to economic demands on the state.

The convergence of disparate philosophical traditions around the concept of citizenship obligations produces a cacophony of critiques about the rights bias and atomism perceived in the social liberalism that informed welfare regimes in affluent English-speaking democracies following the Second World War. These critiques call into question the intellectual foundation of state welfarism in these countries, generating a crisis of legitimation (Cox 1998). In response, there has occurred a rhetorical shift away from a discourse of rights toward one of duties that links eligibility for social entitlements to the fulfillment of social obligations – what S. White (2000) refers to as a shift toward "welfare contractualism." This transition is observed in Canada (for example, Jenson and Saint-Martin 2003), the United States (for example, Mead 1986), Australia (for example, Shaver 2002), New Zealand (for example, Larner 2000), the United Kingdom (for example, Lister 1998), as well as continental Europe (Bussemaker 1998), where social democratic and corporatist welfare regime patterns dominate over Anglo-liberal traditions.

Although the rise of duty discourse is evident across political traditions, the New Right has enjoyed the most political success in English-speaking countries by re-emphasizing the language of social obligations. Responding to an era of fiscal austerity, right-of-centre political parties won electoral support in Canada and elsewhere by synthesizing the concept of welfare contractualism with an overarching animosity toward state provision in an effort to dismantle postwar social security systems. Although Pierson (2001) argues that welfare systems cross-nationally have shown considerable resilience in the face of this challenge, more pronounced qualitative restructuring of state architecture cannot be denied in the liberal welfare regime cluster, including in Canada (for example, McBride and Shields 1997).

The term "regime" merits definitional attention in light of its recent appropriation by politicians and pundits preoccupied with the so-called war on terror. Whereas the latter use the term "regime" to refer principally to state leaders and government apparatuses that allegedly support terrorist organizations, the term is used in comparative welfare literature to capture the "combined, interdependent way in which welfare is produced and allocated between the state, market and family" (Esping-Andersen 1999, 34-35). Evers, Pilj, and Ungerson (1994) further refine this triangular definition of "regime" by aligning the concept with a welfare diamond that appends the voluntary sector to Esping-Andersen's state-market-family framework.

Working with this definition, qualitative regime restructuring does not just denote that policy changes since the 1980s have reduced public expenditures. In the Canadian context, the quantitative cutbacks of resources for social services during the 1980s and 1990s were not new, although they often were more dramatic in scope. Citing work by Banting (1982), McBride and Shields (1997, 22) observe that the social benefits institutionalized under the welfare regime after the Second World War were "in constant flux, expanding in some periods and contracting in others." What is distinct about the more recent round of expenditure reductions is their departure from the commitment to postwar welfare services and the distribution of responsibility for social provision across the welfare diamond that this policy framework assumed. McBride and Shields report that, "in the past ... cuts were carried out with the intention that they were 'temporary' and would be restored with the economic recovery" (ibid.). But spending cuts in the 1990s were enacted as part of an emerging paradigm shift in which federal and provincial governments identified a reduced role for the state in welfare provision as a critical element for an adequate postindustrial social policy course. The commitment to reduce the state's role as a central plank of a new platform is particularly evident at the federal level. The Government of Canada (2000, Chapter 3) lists the achievement of a fifty-year low in federal program spending as a share of GDP (at 11.7 percent in 1999-2000) as a key component of federal efforts to restore public fiscal health, solidifying the foundation for a new welfare regime order.

Jenson (1997a) and her many co-authors portray this shift in paradigm in the language of citizenship that has garnered so much influence in normative literature in recent years (see also Jenson and Phillips 1996; Jenson and Saint-Martin 2003; Jenson and Sineau 2001). Jenson (1997a, 631) employs the term "citizenship regime" to refer not only to the "institutional arrangements" and "rules" that "guide and shape state policy," but also to the concepts and assumptions that occupy centre stage in political-cultural thinking, or what she refers to as "understandings" and the "problem definition employed by states and citizens." A shift in citizenship regime, therefore, signals a recoding of the shared ideas and criteria by which issues are recognized as appropriate subject matter for politics, and, thus, a reorganization of the boundaries of political debate. A restructured citizenship regime articulates a new "paradigmatic representation of ... the 'model citizen,' the 'second-class citizen' and the 'non-citizen,'" recasting what these ideal types can legitimately expect of their neighbours, markets, and governments (632). In the light of emerging duty discourses, regime restructuring seeks to shift "the boundaries of the responsibility mix" between points on the welfare diamond (Jenson and Saint-Martin 2003, 81). The contemporary citizenship regime identifies new forms of security that downplay the social safety net in favour of the now familiar trampoline metaphor. This metaphor signals the state's eagerness to bounce citizens from public assistance toward families, the voluntary sector, and especially the market as part of a strategy to assign more responsibility for welfare creation to these social domains.

The success with which the New Right deployed a duty discourse to recalibrate the postwar citizenship regime prompts some critics of neoliberal restructuring to view the concept of welfare contractualism as an attack on the tradition of social citizenship to which T.H. Marshall (1964) gave voice following the Second World War (Roche 1992; Shaver 2002). I wish to challenge this judgment in this book. I argue that the recent convergence in political thought, which treats fulfillment of social obligations as a condition for social entitlement, actually needs to be advanced further to integrate care as a constitutive responsibility and right of social citizenship that binds men as much as women. This development would complement the attention that policy circles presently pay to employment duties and human-capital acquisition by integrating a new analytic dimension concerned with caregiving throughout all social citizenship commitments. The resulting redesign of the social policy blueprint would dramatically help to minimize inequalities suffered by diverse groups of women, while also addressing a number of the most pressing postindustrial socioeconomic trends that are undergirding fiscal challenges which strain modern welfare systems.

There are solid strategic reasons for scholars and political actors critical of the neoliberal paradigm to embrace the duty discourse. The convergence across disparate philosophical traditions in favour of renewed concern for social responsibilities identifies a starting point for what Gramsci (1971) terms a "counterhegemony." Hegemony is the set of processes that generate "the 'spontaneous' consent given by the great mass of the population to the general direction imposed on social life by the dominant fundamental group" (12). A. Hunt (1993, 229) adds that hegemony involves "the production, reproduction, and mobilization of popular consent" to secure the "leadership" and privilege of those who are already dominant. One implication of this view is that a project becomes dominant only if it addresses, even if just partially, "some aspects of the aspirations, interests and ideology of the subordinate groups" (230).

The heightened concern with social duties that different political camps, including feminists, share with the neoliberal paradigm suggests that some notion of welfare contractualism may represent a part of what is appealing about the reigning citizenship discourse to social groups whose less-privileged status it reinforces. Once recognized, this and other points of convergence that I identify in the book provide openings to refashion constitutive elements of the neoliberal hegemony by revealing issues on which the dominant discourse is silent, as well as by introducing new dimensions that effectively transcend the discourse. Thus, the path to replacing the neoliberal paradigm does not lie so much in negating its vision, which partly resonates with much of the citizenry, but in reconstructing it to reprioritize what is currently missing and, therefore, relocate or exhaust problematic elements that are presently dominant. The concern to move beyond the left/right political framework urged by third way proponents (Giddens 1994, 1999, 2000) and new communitarians (Etzioni 1993, 1996) shares some affinity for this strategic insight. At the very least, points of convergence between disparate political traditions mark cornerstones in a foundation for social citizenship from which individuals with diverging viewpoints can identify areas of agreement that make possible the compromises that are necessary for alternative political movements to succeed.

Beyond strategic considerations, a concern to further develop the duty discourse is theoretically important because it builds on the emerging consensus in the literature, which indicates that "most writers believe that an adequate theory of citizenship requires greater emphasis on responsibilities and virtues" (Kymlicka and Norman 1994, 353). In particular, re-emphasis on social obligations is appropriate to respond to the morally hazardous dynamics that accompany gendered systems of social provision present in families, the voluntary sector, markets, and state infrastructure. The moral hazard concept is typically found in the discourse of economists, particularly in respect of public and private insurance systems. It illuminates how policy may provide individuals and firms that are insured against loss with incentives to behave in socially nonoptimal ways by taking less care to prevent that loss than they would in the absence of insurance. In the current political context, this logic principally informs critiques of employment insurance, social assistance, and the so-called welfare wall, which ostensibly erode motivation to engage in paid work. But the logic is just as germane to what Taylor-Goodby (1991, xi-xii) identified over a decade ago as the perverse policy, economic, and cultural "incentives which encourage men to evade a duty to share in the unwaged labour of social care." These perverse incentives are a primary concern of this book.

The veracity of Taylor-Goodby's diagnosis of the gender division of labour and its link to morally hazardous dynamics remains salient today, although his work is relatively silent about the policy implications of his diagnosis. This lack of attention to policy ramifications is consistent with "the timidity with which authors apply their theories of citizenship to questions of public policy," which Kymlicka and Norman (1994, 368) describe as "a striking feature of the current debate" in the literature. Many authors, they report, "focus more on describing desirable qualities of citizens, and less on what policies should be adopted to encourage or compel citizens to adopt these desirable virtues and practices" (Kymlicka and Norman 2000, 7). The result is that "all too often in the citizenship literature" the work reduces to the platitude that society would function better "if people in it were nicer and more considerate" (Kymlicka and Norman 2003, 217).

This book suffers no such timidity. In the final chapters, I advance the concept of "care*fair*," after which the book is titled. Just as many governments employ active labour market and other workfare policies to encourage or compel citizens to discharge their paid work obligations, so we also need a care*fair* policy commitment to encourage or compel citizens who neglect informal care activities to discharge citizenship duties in the domestic domain. Given the persistent patriarchal division of care, the activities of many men are the primary target of a care*fair* policy framework as it seeks to institutionalize an equitable distribution of caregiving across sexes, classes, and ethnic groups. Crossnationally, more governments are cracking down on so-called deadbeat dads to ensure their fulfillment of financial obligations to children (Hobson 2002). But this financial crackdown does not obviously interrogate cultural norms and practices which distance care provision from many social conventions that define fatherhood and masculinity. In response, I argue that a similar level of tenacity must be demonstrated specifically to urge fathers to fulfill more care responsibilities. The policy levers available to achieve this end are the subject of Chapters 8 and 9.

They examine in detail the incentives associated with existing policies and cultural patterns with the intention of boldly addressing how the state should entice men to assume a just share of unpaid care labour in recognition that provision of this care is an important civic virtue and obligation of citizenship.

Any effort to integrate care as an obligation of citizenship must be attuned to the diverging needs and experiences of care provision and receipt that depend on whether the care recipient is a child, a person with a physical or mental disability, a senior citizen, or an able-bodied, psychologically healthy adult. This book singles out care for children as the primary model for exploration, particularly when assessing existing policies and proposing alternatives. Although care for the elderly is and will be a growing social need as the baby boom generation ages and health care reform stalls, a life-course perspective reveals that child care is an especially significant policy problem in regard to the gender division of care. Research shows that the birth of a child pushes many straight couples along a path of neotraditionalism regardless of their intentions or attitudes about gender roles (Zvonkovic et al. 1996). By the time elder care becomes a concern for members of the new sandwich generation, who at some point will care simultaneously for children and parents, domestic care roles are often already established within heterosexual couples.

The choice to examine child care also responds to the political reality that children are one of the few social groups to be condoned as legitimate dependants within the neoliberal paradigm (Brodie 1996, 135). The paradigm's preoccupation with self-reliance has meant that most other dependency on the state is viewed somewhat suspiciously as an indication of personal failure. The demarcation of children from adults under the guise of legitimate dependency has contributed to a neoliberal preference for targeting income-maintenance programs to children, particularly in an effort to combat child poverty. One result of this policy orientation is that it risks theoretically removing children's well-being from the circumstances of their parents or other guardians. I defend against this risk by directing attention to children and child care in the context of the social citizenship needs of adults.

While principally concerned with the gender division of labour that emerges in response to families' child care needs, the policy analysis in the book is far broader than this one issue. Just as the early post-Second World War era acknowledged a symbiotic relationship between economic policy in its Keynesian guise and social policy designed to refashion the inadequate intra-war social security system, so we again live in an era where there is potential to re-initiate a virtuous circle between economic and social policy. Specifically, I will argue that some measures designed to mitigate systemic gender inequalities and foster work-family balance are necessary to remedy ailments in modern labour markets more generally. Problems that I examine include the looming labour shortage that is anticipated from the warped population pyramid, polarization in the paid hours that people work and the resulting earnings inequality and un(der)employment, as well as declining real wages for young workers, especially men.

The ambition to articulate principles by which to reshape the overarching framework for Canada's social policy blueprint follows in the tradition of two of the most cogent and comprehensive right-of-centre critiques of the Canadian welfare state: Thomas Courchene's (1994a) *Social Canada in the Millennium* and John Richards's (1997) *Retooling the Welfare State,* which were published in partnership with the C.D. Howe Institute. The impressive breadth of policy expertise demonstrated by these authors positions them both to illuminate the manner in which social policy re-emerges in the contemporary context as an indispensable economic factor. As Courchene (1994a, 233) explains, "in an era where knowledge is at the cutting edge of competitiveness, social policy as it relates to human capital and skills formation becomes indistinguishable from economic policy" – a theme he develops further in his subsequent book, *A State of Minds* (2001). Working from this perspective, Courchene and Richards have been important intellectual architects for social policy in Canada over the past decade, exerting particular influence in terms of the delivery of income assistance for children, as well as in respect of the evolution of fiscal federal relations. The federal government's introduction of the Canada Child Tax Benefit and its heightened respect for "competitive federalism" both track policy prescriptions advanced by Richards (1997, Chapter 12 and 243-49) and Courchene (1994a, 154-55, 324; 1997).

The breadth of policy knowledge in their respective treatises is not matched by a similarly strong normative foundation, however. This lacuna is problematic given the ambitious task that Courchene and Richards set for themselves. Courchene (1994a, 3), for instance, begins his book by explaining that its purpose "is to describe, to evaluate, and, ultimately, to redesign Canada's social policy infrastructure ... Given that the manner in which we Canadians decide to rework our social envelope will be one of the defining characteristics of our nation in the twenty-first century, redesigning Social Canada is tantamount to redefining Canada." Invoking Jenson's terminology, Courchene's objective is no less than the redefinition of the country's citizenship regime. But this project does not just require policy expertise. It also demands philosophical inquiry about the kind of society we ought to live in by raising questions of justice, including the requirements of social inclusion, the scope and kinds of inequality we will permit, and so on. The assumptions about these issues that underpin Courchene's alternative vision are, therefore, critical and merit more attention than he provides.

Richards is more attentive than Courchene to normative issues. His analysis includes a careful examination of the philosophical framework of the "Traditional Left," which parented the welfare state in Canada in its first decades. But, like Courchene, Richards does not provide a comparable discussion of the normative framework that guides his own vision for a welfare system appropriate for the postindustrial context. One result, we will see, is that both authors defend social policy blueprints that retain vestiges of what Pateman (1988) referred to as the patriarchal "sexual contract," which is a historical foundation of the liberal philosophical tradition within which the two men work.

Illuminating the patriarchal character of the dominant vision of social citizenship in Canada that Courchene and Richards represent is a key objective of this book. My approach to the subject of social policy redesign thus departs from their methodology by embracing a much stronger concern to merge normative theory from political science, philosophy, sociology, and law with public policy analysis. This approach does not fit the quantitative/qualitative framework through which much policy work is categorized. Nor does the policy work follow in the path of rational choice scholars, power resource theory, or one of the many brands of institutionalism. Instead, policy research in this book is the progeny of the citizenship theorists whom Kymlicka and Norman note have so far been hesitant to enter the foray of policy analysis. It aims to provide an example of the value of expanding public policy scholarship to include theorists as key partners in the world of practical policy review and design.

The normative framework I employ in Care*fair* is unabashedly feminist. Although issues of caregiving now receive attention from third way scholars such as Giddens (1999, 2000) and Esping-Andersen (1999, 2002), new communitarians like Etzioni (1993, 1996), and social conservative organizations, including the Canadian group REAL Women, it remains a uniquely feminist endeavour to treat care as a lens of analysis for citizenship and social policy. As Daly and Lewis (1998, 4) remark, "care is one of the truly original concepts to have emerged from feminist scholarship, and it has served as a central hinge in thinking about how welfare states are or can be gendered. The origins of the concept lie in an attempt to define in its own right the work that makes up caring for others and to analyze how that work reinforced the disadvantaged position of women. Over time, however, the labour focus came to be complemented by a consideration of the wider notion of the social (societal) division of caring and the state's role therein."

The analysis developed in this book is the product of third wave feminism, which resists the hyphenated feminisms of the past. Rather than aligning my analysis with liberal-feminism, socialist-feminism, or communitarian-feminism, the book is better located in feminist literature in terms of its reliance on three fundamental internal debates. The first is research initiated by Gilligan's (1982) work on the ethic of care. The second is literature associated with Pateman's (1989, 179-209) presentation of the limited citizenship options available to women in her discussion of Wollstonecraft's dilemma, especially the ensuing research by Fraser (1994), who articulates the universal caregiver model of postindustrial welfare to transcend this dilemma. The third debate is captured by Collins (1991, 1994), who cogently argues for the experiences of women of colour to be placed at the centre of feminist theorizing and policy research. Readers who are less familiar with feminist scholarship can rest assured that the meaning and significance of these streams of literature will become clear in the following chapters.

Over the course of the analysis, I draw upon insights from these feminist debates to evaluate the ideological deployment of duty discourses in liberal welfare regimes. The intention is to defend a heretofore undeveloped pillar for Canada's social policy framework that would accord far more value to remedying the gender division of labour by obliging men to care, while also acknowledging that private time for domestic care is a necessary condition for social inclusion. The pillar I envision is, therefore, called on to support a balancing act that rejects outright the patriarchal distribution of care without condemning the activity of care itself. The care*fair* vision expects and demands men to care more in order to minimize gender inequality, including inequality in income, participation in the labour market, and access to political power. But this expectation should not be viewed as the imposition of some punishment or hardship on diverse groups of men. The feminist debates that inform this book are explicit that caregiving often is a source of great pleasure, fulfillment, and identity – a source from which the breadwinner model of male citizenship has historically marginalized many men. Thus, not only does care*fair* challenge patriarchy, but it also embraces the potential for public policy to minimize barriers that some men encounter in accessing and cultivating their spheres of affectivity.

In the process, the care*fair* concept casts doubt on visions of social citizenship that equate welfare predominantly with income level, market participation, and human capital. Citizens ought not to be counted as full members of society just by virtue of their affluence, employment, or skills. The time citizens must allocate to secure these goods is also an important consideration because long hours in the labour force or in training often confront citizens with a time crunch that requires them to sacrifice participation in other important areas of social life, including participation in their private networks of intimate, familial, and friendship relations. Care*fair* responds to this risk by suggesting a more nuanced vision of welfare that integrates a richer appreciation for the value that care provision and receipt contribute to individual and group well-being, all the while grappling with the risk that time poverty may constrain citizens' capacities to balance caring with earning.

Organization of the Book

Following this introduction, the book begins in Chapter 2 by returning to the tradition of citizenship defined in seminal social liberal texts by T.H. Marshall (1964) and John Rawls (1971). This starting point is important for three reasons. The first is that the language of social citizenship is relatively foreign to Canadians who are not familiar with the social sciences. In Canada, citizenship is primarily spoken of only in terms of immigration. This observation stands despite the fact that D. White (2003, 58) claims that "*social* citizenship became the most distinctive dimension of Canada's citizenship regime ... well into the 1980s" because of our country's preoccupation with the social programs, especially health care, that distinguish us from our US neighbours. While White's insight may be accurate, the reality is that the distinction citizens observe between domestic and American social policy is not formally named in Canadian parlance; at least it is not regularly spoken of in the language of social citizenship. Thus, for a Canadian audience, it is necessary to return to key conceptual architects of the idea of social citizenship to unpack its meaning and reveal its radical potential.

The focus on Marshall and Rawls is also important because of their strong liberal intellectual heritage. The stickiness of public policy, to which institutionalist scholars concerned with path dependency have alerted social science disciplines, obliges policy analysts to engage with pragmatic politics. Esping-Andersen (1999, 173) captures this theme by noting that "any blueprint for reform is bound to be naïve if it calls for a radical departure from existing welfare regime practice." His subsequent argument "that optimizing welfare in a postindustrial setting will, none the less, require radical departures" signals the challenge that reformists face (ibid.). I propose to tackle this challenge in part by returning to the literature of liberal thinkers like Marshall and Rawls, who defined the intellectual environment that nourished the postwar welfare state in Anglo-liberal regimes like Canada. Policy proposals that demonstrate some consistency with this liberal philosophical heritage are more likely to appeal in the Canadian policy arena than are simple exhortations to import the Scandinavian model.

Finally, it is helpful to re-examine the work of Marshall and Rawls because it is assumptions implicit in their thinking that are a principal target of the duty discourses found across disparate schools of political thought. Traditional liberal assumptions about autonomy, individualism, and rights represent key issues of concern for commentators who worry about a decline of civic virtues in Western societies and a corresponding growth in egoism. Put somewhat differently, renewed emphasis on social obligations represents a citizenship regime shift in Canada because it is replacing the shared assumptions of social liberals like Marshall and Rawls. The restructuring that has occurred in Canada is, thus, only fully appreciated if we assess the political-cultural order that is eroding.

Once the target of the duty discourse is presented, the analysis proceeds by engaging with the newfound attention to social responsibilities given by Courchene and Richards in their respective visions for social citizenship in Canada. Their invocation of the duty concept is consistent with scholarship from five distinct political-ideological camps: neoliberalism, to which I also refer sometimes as economic conservatism; social conservatism, particularly in its neofamilial guise; communitarianism; the third way; and feminism. Chapter 3 is largely descriptive, summarizing the manner in which the first four of these different schools of thought invoke the concept of social responsibility. The renewed concern with social obligations as a leading normative concept in political discourse is presented in the context of the history of citizenship traditions, reflecting the resurgence of themes typical of civic republicanism. This tradition emphasizes active over passive visions of citizenship, which I argue merit further attention and refinement if we wish to embrace care as a constitutive element of citizenship.

Chapters 4 and 5 assess what is right and wrong respectively with each political camp's version of the duty discourse. I draw extensively upon the feminist literatures associated with the work of Gilligan and

Pateman in these evaluations, particularly in regard to the fundamental ambivalence these literatures reveal about caregiving as both a site of rich reward and a deep source of discrimination. This ambivalence motivates the need to develop a policy blueprint that accommodates the finding that caregiving can be a practice that is inherently valuable both socially and privately, but which ultimately requires redistribution within the welfare diamond and across sexes, classes, and ethnic groups in order to minimize discrimination. The analysis lends further support for promoting male obligations to care as well as women's employment responsibilities so long as this promotion unfolds within a policy context that enhances social entitlements to services and programs that facilitate work-family balance.

Chapter 6 addresses in more detail a principal failing of the duty discourses. The problem is the largely one-sided "workerist" approach to social inclusion that they imply, in which paid employment is portrayed as the badge of genuine social inclusion at the expense of participation in other equally important areas of social life, including the domestic sphere. In response, I argue that time for care in one's domestic spaces is an essential element of social belonging that has yet to be fully appreciated by contemporary theorists of inclusion. In this view, obstacles to participation in one's network of intimate, friendship, and familial relations are just as much impediments to the practices of full social membership as are barriers to inclusion in the labour market. This position represents another take on the slogan "The personal is political," which motivates feminist critiques of the public/private divide. I argue that the domestic sphere, which is often viewed as the most private of citizenry spaces, must be treated as a critical sociopolitical domain for the purposes of promoting social inclusion.

The support I offer for this position draws on work advanced by feminist theorists associated with the literature of Patricia Hill Collins. Collins (1991, 1994) demonstrates that motherhood factors significantly in identity politics and issues of individual and collective power. But these themes are often overlooked in social debate when the mothering experiences of women of colour are marginalized in the analysis, including in feminist theorizing. In response, she calls on feminists to reconstruct the dominant view of motherhood in a manner that embraces the circumstances of ethnic minority women. Chapter 6 contributes to this reconstruction process.

Ultimately, though, it is fatherhood more than motherhood that is the target of reconstruction in this book. The rapid rise in female participation in the labour force reflects how the cultural ideal of motherhood has expanded to include paid work expectations and aspirations. This expansion is due in part to women's need to sustain household incomes as a result of the declining real earnings of men since the 1970s. The institution of fatherhood has not kept pace with this postindustrial change, however. It retains strong links to the male breadwinner role to the exclusion of male caregiving, notwithstanding the politically correct, gender-neutral rhetoric that typically accompanies discussions of caring and earning in policy circles and political forums. Following Fraser (1994), I, therefore, argue that the most pressing citizenship innovation requires the reorganization of social policy to induce far more men to modify their behaviour and attitudes to become more like most women today – people who shoulder considerable primary care work in addition to other citizenry obligations and ambitions.

Chapters 7 and 8 conclude the book by exploring the policy changes that are necessary to achieve this cultural transformation. Chapter 7 develops the concept of care*fair* as a cultural analogue to workfare. The objective is to identify and institutionalize policy incentives that will reorganize the existing context of choice that privileges many men economically as a result of their socially sanctioned irresponsibility for caregiving. The chapter also recognizes that some men may be socially excluded from enjoying fully the rewards that can be associated with care provision.

Chapter 8 locates the proposed policy measures designed to minimize the patriarchal division of care in a much broader policy framework under the rubric of what I term the politics of time. Among other issues, this politics interweaves gender equality strategies into a policy tapestry concerned with labour supply, the polarization in earnings, a shift in poverty from the elderly to families with young children, waning fertility, and the rise in time stress reported by Canadians, particularly women. The scope of the analysis points to the value of broadening the analytic boundaries typically associated with the concept of work-family balance to capture a more diverse range of policy issues. In this manner, the discussion shares an affinity with the child-centred social investment strategy and new gender contract recently argued for by Esping-Andersen (2002) and other third way proponents. Ultimately, however, the proposed politics of time distances itself from Esping-Andersen's new welfare vision because his work accommodates primarily those aspects of feminist analysis that pose the least challenge to the male model of citizenship and remains resistant to elements of feminist research that require a more dramatic departure from androcentric assumptions. The analysis in Chapter 8 is also explicitly strategic in tone, conceding that gender equality does not appear to be a primary motivation for dramatic policy departures in the current context. While the book in no way implies that the pursuit of gender equality is only instrumentally valuable, it proposes to capitalize on policy blueprints that represent a win-win strategy for gender justice and other socioeconomic policy envelopes that presently enjoy more political appeal.

2
The American Express™ Model of Citizenship: The Social Liberal Tradition

The "explosion of interest" in citizenship observed by Kymlicka and Norman (1994, 352; 2000, 5) produced a still-burgeoning literature that examines the implications of the concept's social dimension (for example, Barbalet 1988; King and Waldron 1988; Mead 1997a; Orloff 1993; Roche 1992). One striking feature of this literature is that relatively little effort is made to define the terms "social citizenship" and "social rights" other than by identifying these concepts with the welfare state (Adriaansens 1994; Roche 1992). Work by Rees (1995, 314) exemplifies this trend especially well. He assumes that the "notion of a specifically 'social' citizenship ... has a relatively precise and uncontroversial meaning if it is taken to refer to access to, and utilisation of, the bundle of public services conventionally held to make up the modern welfare state."

While its connections to state welfarism are intimate, social citizenship refers in part to a political ideal that is conceptually distinct from the institutional practices that give it de facto power. This distinction is important given that more than two decades of neoliberal restructuring in Canada and elsewhere raise concerns that policy changes have institutionalized weaker commitments to social citizenship than those of the postwar paradigm they replaced. In addition, the tendency to equate citizenship's social element with the welfare state aligns the former predominantly with the goal of income security that Esping-Andersen (1990) documents as a primary focus of postwar welfare states. This alignment risks neglecting other aspects of social citizenship's emancipatory potential, which policy makers were less able or willing to institutionalize in the first decades following the Second World War.

This chapter contributes to remedying the lack of precision with which social citizenship is defined. I return to texts written by two leading twentieth-century theorists who fundamentally shaped postwar scholarship about the subject from within the tradition of social liberalism:

T.H. Marshall's (1964, 65-122) essay "Citizenship and Social Class" and John Rawls's (1971) *A Theory of Justice.* We will see that the liberal vision developed in these texts aligns citizenship's social dimension with the socioeconomic preconditions required for freedom. Three themes receive particular attention: social security, substantive equality of opportunity, and a robust understanding of full community membership that calls for institutional redesign to facilitate dignified inclusion.

The chapter focuses principally on the early texts of Marshall and Rawls, and purposely sets aside Rawls's (1993) later work, *Political Liberalism,* to identify specific assumptions that characterize the paradigmatic approach to theorizing social citizenship in the first three decades following 1945. Familiarity with this approach is necessary to anticipate and understand the various critiques of postwar welfare that are manifest in the duty discourses which have since emerged cross-nationally. Returning to the two seminal texts also allows us to canvass their many insights to determine what elements of the social liberal tradition remain valuable for guiding the development of an alternative postindustrial social citizenship framework in later chapters.

Although the development of the social citizenship concept in Anglo-capitalist welfare states owes considerable debt to many thinkers, including Keynes, Beveridge, Titmuss, and Marsh, the texts by Marshall and Rawls offer particularly rich starting points for defining more precisely the concept's meaning. Notwithstanding criticisms that his work is British-centric (Mann 1987) and patriarchal (Bussemaker and Voet 1998, 287-88; Knijn and Kremer 1997, 331; Sainsbury 1996, 36), Marshall's essay is the central reference point for the academic investigations of citizenship that have dominated normative political theorizing in recent years (Kymlicka and Norman 1994, 2003). His essay also significantly influenced the work of Esping-Andersen (1990), whose interest in decommodification motivated the dominant approach to comparative welfare regime analysis in the 1990s.

Similarly, Rawls's work was the point of focus in the principal debates of Anglo-American political philosophy before the advent of the current focus on citizenship. The evolution from arguments for and against Rawlsian theories toward analyses of citizenship was not accidental. As Shafir (1998, 2) remarks, "John Rawls's systematic revision of the theory of liberal individualism ... helped give the issues we associate with citizenship pride of place in current intellectual and political debates." His work has since been approached by some scholars, notably King and Waldron (1988), as an extensive discussion of what it means to be a citizen or full member of a given society.

My decision to rely on the texts of Marshall and Rawls is also a methodological one. Since their notoriety extends well beyond the disciplinary boundaries within which they write – Marshall as a sociologist and Rawls as a philosopher – their works have been assessed, lauded, and critiqued by scholars from diverse academic backgrounds and have become foundational pieces for theorists from varied intellectual pursuits. The texts' resulting common commodity status marks an accessible starting point from which to initiate an interdisciplinary study of citizenship that builds upon, and puts in dialogue, the insights of political scientists, sociologists, economists, legal theorists, and philosophers.

Seeing the "Social" in Citizenship

Citizenship identifies far more than nationality or ownership of a passport, things with which it is often associated in the vernacular of North Americans. More fundamentally, citizenship articulates the terms of belonging in a society by defining the entitlements and obligations that accompany full membership. Foundational institutions like the constitution and the principal economic and social arrangements in a society engender and enforce citizenry rights and responsibilities that regulate individual participation in and across domestic, market, civic, and political spaces, while also setting constraints on state power. Although the community at issue is most often the nation-state, the language of citizenship is increasingly used to discuss membership in supranational political entities such as the European Union, as well as membership in subnational communities such as the Québécois and Aboriginal groups in light of their aspirations for sovereignty.

T.H. Marshall's approach to citizenship scholarship was particularly innovative because his institutional analysis divided the content of citizenship into three (potential) parts: civil, political, and social (Marshall 1964, 71-72). He associates the civil element with "the rights necessary for individual freedom" that are protected by the court system and the rule of law (71). These institutions provide a basis for "liberty of the person, freedom of speech, thought and faith, the right to own property and to conclude valid contracts, and the right to justice" (ibid.). The political element is concerned with "the right to participate in the exercise of political power" that emerged with the development of parliamentary institutions, including local councils and the democratic electoral system (72). Finally, he links the social element of citizenship with the twentieth-century welfare state, especially the onset of universal education and social security systems. These welfare institutions, he reports, have the potential to give rise to a broad series of citizenry entitlements, ranging "from the right to a modicum of economic welfare and security to the right to share to the full in the social heritage and to live the life of a civilized being according to the standards prevailing in the society" (ibid.).

By distinguishing the three elements, Marshall (1964, 91) teaches that citizenship is inadequately theorized if only its formal legal dimension is appreciated. The opportunity to participate fully in society and to affect its political decisions is not merely a question of the range of political and civil rights that empowers members. Equality before the law does not guarantee all persons the practical ability to invoke and benefit from legal entitlements since unequal social and economic conditions limit, for some, the opportunities to exercise their civil and political liberties (88). As Marshall eloquently puts it:

> Civil rights ... confer [only] the legal capacity to strive for things one would like to possess but do not guarantee the possession of any of them. A property right is not a right to possess property, but a right to acquire it, if you can, and to protect it, if you can get it. But, if you ... explain to a pauper that his property rights are the same as those of a millionaire, he will probably accuse you of quibbling. Similarly, the right to freedom of speech has little real substance, if from lack of education, you have nothing to say that is worth saying, and no means of making yourself heard if you say it. But these blatant inequalities are not due to defects in civil rights, but to lack of social rights. (ibid.)

Thus, of the three elements of citizenship, Marshall is principally concerned with the social dimension, particularly its effects vis-à-vis the tendency for laissez-faire capitalist economies to produce substantial vertical stratification within societies. While civil and political rights are essential to citizenship in a democratic state, his point is that their formal status may mean little to citizens who suffer either "class prejudice and partiality" or the "unequal distribution of wealth" that leaves them bereft of the resources necessary to pursue goals freely, access property, and participate politically (Marshall 1964, 88-91). For Marshall, the urgency of demands generated by need and the unequal status associated with poverty radically undermine the conditions necessary for successful market and political participation, thereby distorting both the contribution that individuals can make and the ends they can achieve. In addition, he observes that the formal status of civil entitlements may render self-perpetuating the social exclusion that results from material constraints. Civil rights have historically been used to deny individuals social protection from the inequalities of a capitalist economy on the grounds that such rights empower citizens to engage in the competitive market equipped with the means to protect themselves (87).

The socioeconomic preconditions for liberty are also a prominent theme in Rawls's work, as is manifest in the lexical ordering of the principles of justice recommended by his renowned thought experiment of the original position (1971). Rawls asks us to imagine the principles that we would select to regulate our claims against one another and to define the governing charter for our society if we were to choose in advance from behind a veil of ignorance, before we knew anything about our community, our social status, intelligence, or life goals. According to Rawls, contractors in this original position would choose two principles. The first would guarantee "each person ... an equal right to the most extensive basic liberty compatible with a similar liberty for others" (Rawls 1971, 60). This principle, he explains, defines and secures "the equal liberties of citizenship," which are, roughly speaking, those identified by Marshall as civil and political rights, such as "political liberty (the right to vote and to be eligible for public office) together with freedom of speech and assembly; liberty of conscience and freedom of thought; freedom of person along with the right to hold (personal) property; and freedom from arbitrary arrest and seizure as defined by the concept of the rule of the law" (61). For Rawls, these basic rights define the terms on which members of a society are equal regardless of whatever social and economic inequalities may otherwise be sanctioned in a community.

Rawls's second principle is concerned with the distribution of wealth and income, identifying the sorts of financial inequalities that are inimical to a genuine commitment to the equal liberties of citizenship. This principle has two parts. The first maintains that "positions of authority and offices of command must be accessible to all" (Rawls 1971, 61). The second part, what Rawls terms the "difference principle," states that inequalities of wealth and income "are just if and only if they work as part of a scheme which improves the expectations of the least advantaged members of society" (75). Inequalities in the distribution of material goods that undermine equal opportunity or otherwise render the least advantaged worse off than they would have been under conditions of strict equality are, therefore, proscribed in Rawls's theory of justice.

Rawls is explicit that the two principles "are to be arranged in serial order with the first principle prior to the second" (1971, 61). Shafir (1998, 7) interprets this arrangement to mean that "once basic liberties, or what [Marshall called civil and political] citizenship rights, are safe-guarded, the rights of the least advantaged, or their social citizenship rights, should be our main consideration in contracting for a just society." But this interpretation does not fully appreciate Rawls's concern for the social element of citizenship. This element is not an afterthought for Rawls but instead a necessary condition for basic liberty. The serial order of the two principles, Rawls (1971, 43) explains, "means ... that the basic structure of society is to arrange the inequalities of wealth and authority in ways consistent with the equal liberties" of civil and political citizenship. The distribution of material resources must be organized in this way since some allocations are fundamentally incompatible with equal liberties and opportunities for all. "Until the basic wants of individuals can be fulfilled, the relative urgency of their interest in liberty cannot be firmly decided in advance" (543, see also 204-5). As Jackman (2000, 243) notes, "it requires little imagination to question the value and meaning of a right to freedom of conscience and opinion without adequate food; to freedom of expression without adequate education; to security of the person without adequate shelter and health care." Accordingly, Rawls concurs with Marshall that a genuine commitment to freedom entails commitments to the social preconditions for liberty – commitments that make up the domain of citizenship's social dimension. Only under "favourable circumstances" are citizens free to prioritize their "fundamental interest in determining [their] life plan" according to their personal talents, values, and objectives (Rawls 1971, 543).

The attention that Marshall and Rawls give to the social and economic context necessary for citizens to effectively exercise civil and political rights is in keeping with a long-standing Western tradition of theorizing citizenship. King and Waldron (1988, 425-26) observe that "Aristotle, Machiavelli, Burke, de Tocqueville, Mill and, in the twentieth century, Hannah Arendt ... have believed that in order to be a citizen of a *polis*, in order to be able to participate fully in public life, one needed to be in a certain socioeconomic position ... People, it was said, could not act as citizens at all, or could not be expected to act well in the political sphere and to make adequate decisions, unless some attention was paid to matters of their wealth, their well-being and their social and economic status."

Marshall and Rawls diverge from many earlier historical figures, however, in terms of the conclusion they draw about the connection between socioeconomic context and the capacity to participate in one's community effectively. While Aristotle, Machiavelli, Burke, and others used this link to ground an argument for restricting citizenship to those who occupy a "suitable" social location, Marshall and Rawls draw the opposite conclusion. The social liberal philosophy urges that social institutions should be arranged so they ensure all members of a society occupy the socioeconomic position in which, the legacy of Western intellectual scholarship about citizenship provides good reason to believe, citizens ought to reside.

The commitment to an ideal of equality among individuals reflects the extraordinary appeal of the liberal tradition, which embraces the egalitarian view that all members of a community count for one and no more than one. Marshall (1964, 87-88) attributes the development of this modern liberal notion of Western citizenship to the shift away from societal practices premised on the differential "status" or honour "associated with class, function and family" toward practices that presumed contracts "between men who are free and equal in status." Taylor (1994) has developed this theme, identifying the social transition with the emergence of the modern notion of dignity. Since "honour" offers a primary societal organizing principle that is incompatible with the onset of democracy, Taylor observes that the politics of honour was inevitably superseded by the politics of "equal dignity" or "equal citizenship" (27). We use the term "dignity" today, he explains, "in a universalist and egalitarian sense, where we talk of the inherent 'dignity of human beings,' or of citizen dignity" (ibid.).

The politics of equal dignity maintains that all human beings are equally worthy of respect because of a universally shared potential. Taylor (1994, 41) and others credit the philosopher Kant with being one of the first to articulate this idea. According to Kant (1993, 434-35), we all possess dignity and should be treated with respect as intrinsically valuable ends in ourselves, rather than as means to some end, by virtue of our common status as rational agents who have the potential to direct our lives in reference to moral principles. Although the detailed definition of dignity may have changed, Taylor (1994, 41) remarks that something like Kant's evocation of the concept has become the basis for our intuitions about equal citizenship. Most notably, the politics of dignity continues to direct our attention to some universal potential or capacity that all humans share regardless of our differences. "This potential, rather than anything a person may have made of it, is what ensures that each person deserves respect. Indeed, our sense of the importance of potentiality reaches so far that we extend this protection even to people who through some circumstance that has befallen them are incapable of realizing their potential in the normal way – handicapped people, or those in a coma, for instance" (41-42).

A Three-Part Framework for Social Citizenship

Independently of one another, Marshall and Rawls both align the social element of citizenship with a three-part framework that would entrench state commitments to (i) social security, (ii) substantive equality of opportunity, and (iii) dignified community membership. In terms of security, Rawls (1971, 87) advocates the concept of a guaranteed "reasonable social minimum," one that can be calculated in terms of the material resources of the more privileged in society so that "the advantages of the better situated improve the condition of the least favored." Marshall (1964) anticipates this idea, calling for a system of social services that creates both "a universal right to real income which is not proportionate to the market value of the claimant" (96) and a "guaranteed minimum ... supply of certain essential goods and services (such as medical attention and supplies, shelter and education)" (101). In Marshall's view, such a system of social services has the potential to effectively counter the tendency for capitalist economies to commodify citizens. The "real income" on which citizens depend for their survival and well-being would no longer be contingent on the sale of their labour power for a wage that makes little reference to their "social needs and status" as citizens (80).

The endorsement that Marshall and Rawls give a guaranteed minimum reflects a commitment to an egalitarian foundation for society. As Marshall (1964, 102) puts it, the social liberal concern is the "general enrichment of the concrete substance of civilized life." This enrichment demands a "general reduction of risk and insecurity" premised on an equalization of social conditions "between the more and the less fortunate at all levels – between the healthy and the sick, the employed and the unemployed, the old and the active, the bachelor and the father of a large family" (ibid.).

However, the commitment to an egalitarian foundation by no means implies a commitment to absolute equality of outcomes. Rather, consistent with Rawls's two principles of justice, the social liberal emphasis is upon strict legal equality matched by broader commitments to foster equality of opportunity. The latter may ultimately result in inequalities of income and other material conditions among citizens as they pursue disparate opportunities that generate different material rewards.

In Rawls's work, the commitment to securing equal opportunity is a substantive one – not merely a formal one. This distinction indicates that positions in a society should not only be "open to talents ... in a formal sense," but, as Rawls (1971, 73) argues, citizens also "should have a fair chance to attain [those talents]." In a just society, he explains, it is essential that "the expectations of those with the same abilities and aspirations should not be affected by their social class" (ibid.). Thus, Rawls concludes, "free market arrangements must be set within a framework of political and legal institutions which regulates the overall trends of economic events and preserves the social conditions necessary for fair equality of opportunity" (ibid.).

Marshall expresses an equally robust commitment to substantive equality of opportunity in the context of education policy. A public commitment to education, he argues, is critical to prevent cyclical privilege premised on intergenerational inheritance and is also a cornerstone for "the right to equality of opportunity" (1964, 109). But the right to equal opportunity is ultimately "an instrument of social stratification" (110). Public provision of education, he claims, guarantees "the equal right to display and develop differences, or inequalities; the equal right to be recognized as unequal. In the early stages of the establishment of such a system the major effect is, of course, to reveal hidden equalities – to enable the poor boy to show that he is as good as the rich boy. But the final outcome is a structure of unequal status fairly apportioned to unequal abilities" (109).

In Marshall's view, education policy, and social citizenship more generally, do not combat inequality per se; they combat illegitimate inequality. Democratic citizenship, he suggests, is entirely consistent with "status differences ... provided they do not cut too deep ... and provided they are not an expression of hereditary privilege" (1964, 116). Inequalities are tolerable so long as they "are not dynamic" and, thus, do not foster an institutional setting that structures opportunities which for all intents and purposes are unavailable to some because of their socioeconomic starting points.

Preoccupied with the tension between social citizenship and capitalist markets, Marshall's acknowledgment of legitimate social inequality suggests that the two social forces can co-exist: one must not inevitably succumb to the other. Despite his much-quoted claim that "in the twentieth century, citizenship and the capitalist class system have been at war" (1964, 84), Marshall's qualification that "the phrase is rather too strong" better reflects his overarching analysis of the relationship (110). For Marshall, citizenship "impose[s] modifications" on capitalism, but markets must still function within limits (ibid.). There remains a functional reciprocity between state and capitalist market, since the latter powers the economic growth necessary to enrich citizenship status with social security that can be distributed fairly among all members of society.

Thus, in keeping with his contemporaries Keynes and Beveridge, the postwar social and economic strategy advocated by Marshall is one of embedded liberalism – the combination of economic liberalization with a robust commitment to social protection and inclusion (see also Roche 1992, 22).

In addition to security and equal opportunity, a third theme is present throughout Marshall's and Rawls's discussions of the socioeconomic preconditions for liberty: the theme of dignified social membership. The thought experiment of the original position with which Rawls describes and defends a social order to which citizens would voluntarily consent can be read as an examination of what it means to be a citizen or a full member of a society. King and Waldron (1988, 439-40) develop this point, arguing that the social contract tradition that Rawls employs carefully distinguishes between an individual's status as a subject of a community and his or her status as a genuine citizen:

> A person is a mere *subject* of a regime and not a citizen, if its rules and policies will be applied to him or her whether he or she likes it or not and whether they serve his or her interests or not. They are applied without reference to his or her consent. But, since Locke, the liberal tradition has always been that we should try and think of subjects as though they were founding members of the society in which they live. Even though they cannot actually choose the regime they live under, nevertheless in our attempts to evaluate and to legitimize such a regime, we should at least ask what sort of order they would have chosen if they had had the choice. This is the tradition Rawls pursues. For Rawls, being a member of a society is not just a matter of living in and being subject to a social framework, it is also a matter of how that framework is justified.

This approach to reading *A Theory of Justice* suggests an interpretation of Marshall's (1964, 84) view that "citizenship is a status bestowed on those who are full members of a community." Integral to the notion of citizenship that runs throughout Rawls's (1971, 15) project is the "intuitive idea ... that since everyone's well-being depends upon a scheme of cooperation without which no one could have a satisfactory life, the division of advantages should be such as to draw forth the willing cooperation of everyone taking part in it, including those less well situated." This position implies that individuals are self-respecting full members of a community if and only if it can reasonably be expected that they would voluntarily "collaborate with" those "better endowed, or more fortunate in their social circumstances" (103). Rawls's difference principle in turn suggests terms under which it is reasonable to expect such participation would be forthcoming: when persons can be assured that society's basic institutional structure is designed to reflect appropriate concern for their needs and interests in addition to those of other members. Appropriate concern is demonstrated, the difference principle implies, when a community endeavours to ensure that no individual loses out while subject to the social order, and that inequalities in wealth and income benefit even those who are least advantaged in the community.

The intuitive idea underlying the difference principle is that we can imagine that parties in the original position initially propose an arrangement in which all social primary goods are distributed equally. Everyone in this case would have similar rights and duties, and all income and wealth would be apportioned identically. "This state of affairs," Rawls (1971, 62) suggests, "provides a benchmark" for judging the relative merit of alternative social arrangements. Should some inequalities of financial resources and organizational powers raise the economic and social well-being of even those least advantaged in society above the hypothetical benchmark, then all contractors in the original position would have reason to accept the inequalities. No party to the initial contract stands to lose from such unequal distributions (assuming that long-term equality of opportunity is not undermined [302-3]), even if he or she winds up in the least privileged social location within the society he or she is co-designing.

The appropriate concern that full members merit under Rawls's scheme closely parallels Marshall's definition of the social element of citizenship. We have seen that Marshall's (1964, 72) definition references a range of entitlements intended to guarantee that citizens lead a civilized life according to the standards of the day. There is nothing in Marshall's work to suggest, as Rawls does, that a guaranteed standard of civilization premised on the tastes and technologies of the time would permit inequalities in wealth and income if and only if they benefit individuals occupying the least privileged positions in society. Nevertheless, Marshall's reference to a standard of civilization complements Rawls by proposing a strict constraint on what inequalities are permissible. This standard rules out inequalities that exceed a point where the *relative* material deprivation that some suffer renders them uncivilized by the standards of their more privileged peers. It also defends against an impoverished vision of citizenship that is content merely to organize basic institutional arrangements to treat the suffering of the less fortunate. One does not lead a civilized life because the state will treat one's poverty with (stigmatized) income assistance or one's illness with medical services if, as J. Bakan (1997, 141) observes, the state simultaneously "supports and enforces social relations largely responsible for causing that suffering, for making people poor and making them sick." Instead, the right to live a civilized life suggests a state duty to ensure that the institutional order does not relegate the "political and economic causes of poverty and illness ... to the so-called private and depoliticised world of biology, individual choice and ability, family and the market" where they "become invisible and irrelevant" (ibid.).

The difference principle and standard of civilization criteria with which Rawls and Marshall respectively align full community membership have radical implications. As Rawls (1971, 87) explains, the institutions presently responsible for redistributing wealth and income "are riddled with grave injustices" and, therefore, require reorganization so that their design ensures "the difference principle is satisfied consistent with the demands of liberty and fair equality of opportunity." Similarly, Marshall's standard of civilization demands the redesign of social institutions that are complicit in reinforcing social relations that sustain individual marginalization and, therefore, impede some community members from accessing the means to achieve personal projects in a socially respected way.

Dwyer (2000, 52) has recently argued against the view that Marshall's vision of social citizenship entails dramatic institutional reordering. In his view, "it would be wrong to attribute to Marshall a more radical agenda; Marshall's citizenship theory fits comfortably within the liberal democratic tradition which seeks to emphasise equality of opportunity and simultaneously make tolerable continuing inequality of outcome by the promotion of universally held rights."

While Dwyer's interpretation would appear misguided in light of the standard of civilization criterion, it does reflect the incomplete way in which many other scholars have drawn on Marshall's work. For instance, the extensive literature spawned by Esping-Andersen's (1990) *The Three Worlds of Welfare Capitalism* focuses almost entirely on the issue of income and social security under the intellectual rubric of "decommodification." More recently, third way scholars such as Giddens (1999, 2000) and Esping-Andersen (2002) have given considerably more attention to equality of opportunity as part of their discussions of the social investment state. In contrast, the standard of civilization with which Marshall aligns dignified community membership has received considerably less attention than the other two themes by which he develops the meaning of social citizenship. As a result, the radical character of Marshall's vision has been muted in the literature, which partly explains Dwyer's analysis. In response, in this book the institutional redesign that is required for dignified community membership will be pushed to the forefront of analysis in subsequent chapters.

Although radical, the institutional restructuring that is urged by the difference principle and the civilization standard is ultimately consistent with the classical liberal preoccupation with economic efficiency. Provided an egalitarian social foundation is secured, Rawls's second principle urges communities to harness the power of capitalist markets (see especially Rawls 1971, 67-75). He indicates that the incentive effects implicit in markets offer societies an opportunity to capitalize on the varied levels of ambition and natural talents among their members and thereby maximize economic growth and the value of available resources. When regulated by a social structure that does not permit inequalities to cut "too deep" or express "hereditary privilege" (Marshall 1964, 116), Rawls (1971, 179) maintains that economic efficiency has the potential to render "the distribution of natural abilities as a collective asset." The "more fortunate" in the lottery of natural talents and ambition prosper more within competitive markets, but in the just society that has undergone institutional recalibration, they do so "in ways that help those who have lost out" (ibid.).

State Welfare

The social liberal concern with institutional redesign reflects Rawls's (1971, 7) assertion that the "primary subject of justice is the way in which the major social institutions distribute fundamental rights and duties and determine the division of advantages from social cooperation." For Rawls, major institutions include "the political constitution ... competitive markets, private property in the means of production and the monogamous family" (ibid.). Interrelationships between these institutions are critical because they generate disparate social locations within a community into which individuals are born. Some of these starting places are more favourable than others, Rawls argues, and the inequalities that result run "especially deep ... Not only are they pervasive, but they affect men's initial chances in life; yet they cannot possibly be justified by an appeal to the notions of merit or desert. It is these inequalities, presumably inevitable in the basic structure of any society, to which the principles of social justice must in the first instance apply" (ibid.).

Some social locations are advantageous because they provide greater access to what Rawls (1971, 62) terms primary social goods: things that every person is presumed to want because they "normally have a use whatever a person's rational plan of life." In a Rawlsian framework, primary social goods include "rights and liberties, powers and opportunities, income and wealth" (ibid.), as well as the conditions required for self-respect (440). These goods are "social" because they are generated, distributed, and regulated by the rules of the major institutions that constitute society's basic structure (92). They are "primary" because they "are necessary means" regardless of one's goals and commitments (93). The more primary social goods one possesses, the more one can be assured of success in carrying out one's intentions, whatever the objectives may be.

Since the distribution of primary social goods profoundly affects individuals' life prospects, Rawls surmises that the job of negotiators in the original position is to establish principles to organize a society's institutional development to distribute them fairly. The parties to the initial contract can be seen as representing a community's (hypothetical) first parliament or senate, albeit one with unique characteristics since decision makers are blinded by the veil of ignorance. Ultimately, it is up to representative individuals in the original position to function as a decision-making body for the community in order to determine the distribution of the privileges or social goods that accompany group membership through their design and organization of the community's major institutions. The thought experiment thus retains pride of place for a governing body in terms of welfare provision, since the constitution, system of property, market, and other institutions are malleable to the agreements that initial legislators make in the original position.

The social liberal preoccupation with state welfare provision also stems from its predominantly class-based analysis of social citizenship, a point of focus that is obvious in Rawls's difference principle, as well as in the title of Marshall's text "Citizenship and Social Class." The postwar paradigm's focus on class has important ramifications for its treatment of the state, market, and households as potential sources of welfare. In particular, Roche (1992, 16, 43) observes that this focal point renders the paradigm susceptible to overemphasizing the social security made available by state services and obscuring the contributions of non-state sources of welfare. This risk arises for two related reasons.

First, class-based analyses have the potential to divert attention from the welfare contributions made predominantly by women within the sphere of private homes. A man of his time, Marshall's primary concern with class takes for granted a patriarchal division of labour and perpetuates a public/private dichotomy that rejects the latter realm as an appropriate subject of theorizing and political evaluation. Consequently, Marshall tends to see women as homemakers and mothers rather than as workers and political actors, despite the extensive wartime evidence to the contrary. This is particularly evident, Roche (1992, 33) reports, in Marshall's formulation of the broad complex of social systems that constitute the modern context of welfare – what Marshall (1981, 123-36) refers to as the "hyphenated society." In his list of systems, Marshall includes the welfare state, democracy, and capitalism but not families. While Roche (1992, 33) notes that Marshall on occasion is sensitive to the important role that families play as "'the original and basic' welfare service," the fact that a key organizing framework for much of his analysis of social citizenship does not reference families speaks volumes.

Rawls also largely ignores the household sphere. As Okin (1989, 94) first noted, by the time Rawls (1971, 303) announces that his "sketch of the system of institutions that satisfies the two principles of justice is now complete," he has examined all of the major institutions that he initially listed under this heading *except* the family. Rawls's disinterest in the domestic sphere, like Marshall's, probably reflects the influence of the public/private dichotomy and the patriarchal division of labour. This influence is evident in Rawls's claim that "we may think of the parties in the original position as heads of families" (128), and in his description of the family "as a small association, normally characterized by a definite hierarchy, in which each member has certain rights and duties" (467). The assumption that negotiators of the initial contract occupy a traditionally male role implies that the status quo within families, and the distribution of labour between the sexes, is taken for granted. In keeping with this implication, Rawls's "first law" of moral psychology presumes that "family institutions are just" (490). This presumption, Okin (1989, 94) remarks, suggests that "families ... must become just in some different way (unspecified by [Rawls]) from other institutions, for it is impossible to see how the viewpoint of their less advantaged members gets to be heard" in the original position.

In addition to downplaying the welfare contributions of diverse groups of women in private households, the dominant postwar paradigm's class-based focus generates a sense of ambivalence toward competitive markets, reserving considerable theoretical room to prioritize state-fostered social security. A class-infused lens is especially likely to portray capitalism, as Marshall (1964, 84) often does, as "a system, not of equality, but of inequality." When so characterized, competitive markets are viewed primarily as forces to dampen, contain, and tame. In response, the dominant paradigm invokes the state to mitigate the vertical stratification produced by capitalist markets through various redistributive practices (Rawls 1971, 73), including a public social security system (87; Marshall 1964, 101). The resulting emphasis on state-delivered welfare risks minimizing the positive contributions of the wage system to the well-being and personal security of paid workers and their dependants.

Roche (1992, 41-42) argues that this risk is exacerbated because the postwar social liberal tradition takes full employment for granted. It acknowledges that a public social security system depends on a successful industrial economy that is highly mechanized and labour intensive. Such an economy not only relieves the state of financial responsibility for potentially unemployed individuals, but also provides the tax base for income security programs and other public spending. However, in keeping with Keynesianism and a commitment to countercyclical macroeconomic measures, the postwar paradigm assumes that the labour market is politically manipulable. Thus, even in contexts when the social liberal paradigm acknowledges the welfare contributions of markets, it elevates the position of the state by assuming that governments can realistically manage and sustain, through full-employment policy, the economic conditions required to produce a tax base for substantial state welfare spending.

The Citizen as Rights Claimer

The preoccupation with the distribution of primary social goods by major institutions renders the social liberal vision of citizenship more passive than active. "Citizenship is a status" in Marshall's (1964, 84) historical analysis. It is not conditional on some form of social participation, but is conferred on full members of a community. This represents what I call the American Express™ model of citizenship. Just as the credit card company's slogan informs customers that "membership has its privileges," so the social liberal emphasizes that community membership comes with privileges – the rights, liberties, powers, opportunities, income, and wealth that institutions distribute. While we will see in successive chapters that social liberalism contemplates the role of social duties in its citizenship vision, the paradigm remains reluctant to impose citizenship obligations that may imply a state preference for specific opinions, values, or modes of action (Bussemaker and Voet 1998, 294). The result is that Rawls and, especially, Marshall advance a view of postwar citizenship that is defined principally in terms of rights and endows the citizen with the status of rights claimer (for example, Kymlicka and Norman 1994, 354). As Roche (1992, 30) observes, the various duties to which the paradigm alludes "are typically either unspoken, relatively muted or underemphasized in relation to its emphasis on the new social *rights of individuals* in the postwar welfare state."

The social liberal preoccupation with citizen entitlements is unsurprising given the dominant paradigm's tendency to focus on state welfare. Citizenship rights typically take the form of legitimate claims on the state. They are the duties (negative or positive) that the state owes its individual members. Thus, when analysis centres on state action, it can be expected that talk of citizenship rights (state duties) is likely to predominate over discussion of the duties that citizens owe one another as individuals or as a collectivity.

The dominant paradigm's preoccupation with citizenship rights, rather than duties, also reflects the historical context within which the modern Western concept of citizenship evolved. As Marshall (1964, 84) indicates, the development of the politics of dignity was premised on the equalization of rights and entitlements between individuals, as well as the enrichment of citizenship status with new types of rights (see also Taylor 1994, 37). By the beginning of the postwar era, the advent of new rights had become a priority among political actors and the general public. There emerged a sense that the citizenry was owed repayment for the discharge of its "national duties of suffering and sacrifices during the Great Depression and the Second World War" (Roche 1992, 31). Given its performance organizing the military effort and regulating the wartime economy, the state was in turn deemed capable of managing the expansion of the public sphere to protect a series of new social rights to security and well-being. Newfound prosperity in the 1950s and 1960s also provided the state with the additional fiscal capacity to deliver the welfare services increasingly demanded by citizens. The postwar welfare consensus was the result. There arose a widely accepted belief among the public that an activist state could resolve the pressing problems of modern society by assuming increased responsibility for welfare-related needs formerly identified as the appropriate domain of private individuals and families (Brodie 1995, 14-15).

The relatively passive character of social liberal citizenship is subject to one important qualification, however. While downplaying social responsibilities, the social liberal tradition accentuates how rights empower the individual to pursue self-selected activities. As Barbalet (1988, 16) explains, rights "attach a particular capacity to persons by virtue of a legal or conventional status. That is, persons may have certain capabilities or opportunities for particular actions – certain powers – as a consequence of their [citizenship] status." The citizen as rights claimer is, thus, the hero of liberal theory, the autonomous individual, who is free to participate in whatever activities he or she desires, provided that this participation does not unduly limit the right and capacity to participate that other full members of the community also enjoy. Although this vision does not require political participation or civic-spiritedness, it nevertheless prioritizes the individual's capacity to be active in some individually chosen domain(s).

Social Liberalism Aligns Autonomy with Individualism

The notion of autonomy that pervades social liberalism is a distinctive and conflicted one. On one hand, we have seen that social liberals are concerned with the preconditions for liberty, which underscore their discussion of the social dimension of citizenship. Their focus on *social* citizenship intimates a view of autonomy that is receptive to the idea of interdependence and that resists aligning agency with individualism. Rawls's (1971, 4) presumption that "society is a cooperative venture for mutual advantage" that "is typically marked by a conflict as well as by an identity of interests" lends support to this interpretation.

On the other hand, however, the majority of analysis in *A Theory of Justice* is cautious about interdependence, and Rawls often favours the language of individualism that is a prominent feature of liberalism more generally. Sandel (1984), for instance, observes that Rawls's original position presupposes an individualist model of personhood that is insensitive to the role that community and relationships play in imbuing citizens with values, life pursuits, and social roles. For the veil of ignorance to operate, Sandel explains, the original position presumes "there is always a distinction between the values I *have* and the person I *am*" (86). To be capable of choice before I know my class or social status, intelligence, physical abilities, interests, or system of values, I must stand to my circumstances always at a certain distance. There must be a subject "me" that is prior to and independent of any ambitions or desires. Regardless of what values or goals I hold, I must be capable of detaching myself to assume an allegedly neutral, unbiased perspective suitable for debating questions of justice.[1] This is the vision of the "unencumbered self."

Implicit in the distinction that Rawls draws between the people we are and the ambitions or values that we hold is an ideal of human agency. If we take Rawls's thought experiment seriously, Sandel (1984, 86) notes that what appears "most essential to our personhood ... [is] not the ends we choose but our capacity to choose them." Prioritization of the capacity to choose reflects the significance of autonomy and independence to our understanding of human agency. Only if my identity is not tied to the aims and interests that I have at any particular moment can I be considered free and capable of genuine choice. Only if I stand at some distance to my circumstances can I regard myself as the subject as well as the object of experience. It is the capacity to transcend my values and pursuits that ensures I am an initiator of action rather than an instrument of the purposes for which I strive.

The unencumbered self thus advances a "liberating vision," one that is often conceived as a model of what is best in human nature (Sandel 1984, 87). Our allegedly essential capacity to choose our values and life-defining projects suggests that at some fundamental level we are unfettered by the dictates of nature and the shackles of social expectations. The distinction between the persons we are and the values we hold portrays human beings as sovereign agents, capable of adopting, and perhaps more importantly resisting, custom, tradition, or inherited status. This capacity to engage with and resist sociocultural expectations enjoys the status of a character ideal in contemporary Western society. Code (1987, 359) observes that the unencumbered self's "mode of being" as a self-originating agent, a self-defining and self-realizing subject, "is considered worthy of admiration and emulation."

However, the typically liberal ideal of the autonomous, self-defining agent rarely ends with recognition of the alleged distance between the persons we are and the values and pursuits that we adopt. Beyond the encumbrances of custom, tradition, and inherited status, the ideal of autonomy associated with the unencumbered self often includes a range of additional characteristics that ostensibly secure our capacities to choose. In particular, Gilligan (1987, 29) observes that liberal theory often "align[s] the self and morality with separation and autonomy – the ability to be self-governing," thereby associating personal relations or caring commitments with "self-sacrifice" or restraints on one's ability to pursue self-selected interests. Similarly, Kymlicka (2002, 419) remarks that much liberal theory "not only presupposes that we are autonomous adults, it seems to presuppose that we are adults *who are not care-givers for dependents.*"

In the original position, this atomistic tendency is most obvious in Rawls's (1971, 13, 127) insistence that initial contractors are "mutually disinterested." Contractors are assumed to be occupied first and foremost with the advancement of their own concerns and "take no interest in one another's interests" except insofar as the pursuit of personal goals requires it. Agents who demonstrate this mutual disinterest have no relations premised (at least in part) on affection or other sentiments that may motivate individuals to prioritize satisfaction of the pursuits of others on a par with, if not above, their own.

Relationships are not entirely absent from Rawls's original position. He describes parties to the initial contract "as heads of families, and therefore as having a desire to further the welfare of their nearest descendants" (1971, 128). But when describing the original position, Rawls does not engage carefully with the patriarchal assumptions implicit in imagining initial contractors as heads of families (Okin 1989, Chapter 5). Nor does his original position carefully consider what genuine concern for one's closest descendants entails on a daily basis, or the potential for that concern to encumber individuals either temporally or psychologically with varied obligations that impede their flexibility to pursue diverse goals. Instead, the depiction of initial contractors as representatives of continuing hereditary lines serves the more limited role for Rawls of explicitly including concern for intergenerational equality in the original position.

Rawls's commitment to mutual disinterestedness in the original position is not intended to rule out the possibility "that once the veil of ignorance is removed, the parties find that they have ties of sentiment and affection" (1971, 129). Foremost among these ties, we can assume, are close family members and other intimate relations whose interests and ends we wish to advance. Nevertheless, for methodological reasons, Rawls excludes motivational factors indexed to feelings of affection for others from deliberations about the initial contract. "At the basis of theory," Rawls explains, "one tries to assume as little as possible" (ibid.). The original position is, therefore, constructed "to incorporate widely shared and yet weak conditions" that do not depend on contentious assumptions (ibid.). Included in the set of assumptions that are subject to controversy, Rawls believes, is the presupposition that a conception of justice rests on extensive ties of natural sentiment between individuals.

By entrenching a commitment to mutual disinterestedness in the original position, Rawls permits a gradual alignment of autonomy with individualism. There is no interdependence recognized in the original position. Indeed, the point of the original position is to establish the terms of future collaboration. Initial contractors at the bargaining table are depicted as self-sufficient individuals willing to concede, if not welcome, a series of new interdependencies to capitalize on the social cooperation that makes possible a better life for all than any one could live by his or her own efforts alone (Rawls 1971, 4). Thus, the starting point for Rawls's thought experiment is a set of autonomous, self-reliant agents who cautiously approach interdependence as an after-thought through the protected mechanism of a contract. The contract establishes a set of rights to protect parties' highly valued independence from the undue intrusion of other (potentially self-serving) individuals who are intent on achieving their own personal goals.

An Ideal against Which to Measure Actual Achievement

The liberating vision of the unencumbered self who is empowered with the rights of social citizenship that Marshall and Rawls defend is an ideal, not a description of reality. Rawls's invocation of the social con-tract concept by no means suggests a society could "be a scheme of cooperation which men enter voluntarily in a literal sense" (1971, 13). Nonetheless, imagining the sort of society that equal people would con-sent to, Rawls argues, provides insights and criteria with which to meas-ure the justness and inclusiveness of existing communities. Indeed, he argues that any society satisfying "the principles which free and equal persons would assent to under circumstances that are fair" would "come as close as a society can to being a voluntary scheme" (ibid.). Marshall (1964, 84) goes further, arguing that the "image of an ideal citizenship" is not just important as a benchmark "against which achievement can be measured"; it is also a vision "towards which aspiration can be directed."

According to the social liberal tradition, a society's actual achieve-ment along the path toward the ideal of equal dignity and social citi-zenship can be measured in terms of its institutional design. The historical analysis that runs throughout Marshall's essay acknowledges that rights have little meaning and influence in the absence of an insti-tutional context capable of enforcing and protecting entitlements on behalf of citizens (see also Barbalet 1988, 6). The de facto content of citizenship status, therefore, depends for Marshall on the history of a society's institutional development. As social institutions evolve, so do the de facto rights of citizenship.

Cross-nationally, social entitlements have never been formalized to the same degree as civil and political rights. Unlike citizenship's other dimensions, social rights do not receive comparable protection under international covenants (Schabas 2000, 199-200), and they "rarely are built into national political constitutions in any full, explicit and unequivocal way" (Roche 1992, 225). Canada's Charter of Rights and Freedoms is an apt example. While the charter alludes to a right to equal opportunity by sanctioning affirmative action programs in section 15(2), it includes no explicit protections against material deprivations that undermine citizens' abilities to participate fully in our cultural, political, and economic spaces. Reflecting the dearth of constitutional protection for social rights, Hirschl (2000) reports that civil rights litigation accounts for the vast majority of charter cases heard in the country, and that the success of civil liberties and negative rights claims is twice that of claims made on the basis of social or collective entitlements. He reports similar trends in New Zealand and Israel.

Lacking formal expression at a constitutional level, social rights are considerably more ambiguous and intangible than are civil and political entitlements in the public eye. As a de facto status, there can be no doubt that social citizenship occupies a less secure footing than its civil and political counterparts. This diminished legal status likely reflects the fiscal conditionality of citizenship's social dimension. The provision of social services and income transfers requires a level of public expenditure not associated with the civil and political rights of modern citizenship (Barbalet 1988, 70-72; Roche 1992, 34-35). Therefore, the full scope of social rights to education and health care is contingent not solely on service delivery infrastructure, but also on a state's institutional capacity to generate revenue (Marshall 1964, 104). Evaluating the extent of this state capacity raises questions about income redistribution between members of a community, including the share of personal or family income that should appropriately be paid to purchase public services and fund income transfers. This line of questioning inevitably confronts concerns about individual property rights. The result is that the social dimension of citizenship exists in continual tension with citizenship's civil element. Given the diverging class affiliations associated with civil and social rights, Marshall (87-88) implies that it is imprudent to assume the state will equally guarantee both dimensions of citizenship. If nothing else, the less formal expression of social rights ensures they are subject to recurrent political contestation, something which neoliberal advocates have capitalized on in recent decades.

The Legitimate Expectations of Citizens Define the Qualitative Content of Social Rights

Setting aside the historical and fiscal factors that explain the less explicit articulation of citizenship's social dimension in a constitutional context, one senses in Marshall's work that this less formalized expression also appropriately reflects the character of social citizenship. Social rights that demand benefits in the form of a service "cannot be precisely defined," Marshall (1964, 104) argues. It is hard to capture a social right's "qualitative element" in the abstract formulation that legislation typically demands. For instance, the full meaning of a right to education is not discernible from legislation that states all children of a certain age will attend school. Rather, its actual meaning is contingent on the educational system's commitment to factors that affect the quality of children's educational experience: classroom size, teacher training, and the educational materials and opportunities made available to students and instructors. Similarly, a right to health insurance may make it possible for every citizen to visit a doctor. But the full impact of that right depends on the health care system's capacity to ensure that individuals' ailments are properly cared for.

Although the qualitative element is difficult to capture in legal documents, Marshall (1964, 104) is adamant that it is this aspect of social rights that matters most to citizens: for instance, what citizens can legitimately expect from a right to health care given their community's socioeconomic context. When the expectations that citizens hold about health care, education, or social insurance are perceived to be reasonable, they may motivate state initiatives in these areas and thereby create obligations on the state. As Marshall (1964, 104) observes, "expectations officially recognized as legitimate ... become ... details in a design for community living."

Marshall does not provide a clear sense of the criteria by which citizenry expectations are granted legitimacy by the state. Given his commitment to the view that social citizenship generates a right to lead a civilized life according to the standards of the day, one might surmise that official recognition is merited by expectations that support social inclusion, equality, dignity, and so forth. Simultaneously, the language of legitimate expectations suggests the concept of social consensus. As more people share expectations, the state may be motivated to consider their positions more carefully. Still, the desire to identify precisely when expectations are legitimate raises questions for which definitive answers are infrequent. Broad agreement alone cannot be a sufficient criterion of legitimacy since members of patriarchal, racist, or homophobic communities may widely share expectations that are entirely unjust and illegitimate. What is more, citizenry expectations (legitimate or otherwise) will change over time in response to economic growth, technological advances, and ideological shifts and, therefore, will forever be a subject of ongoing negotiation between competing stakeholders. Indeed, this dynamic quality is what renders it difficult to formally express in a constitutional context the qualitative dimension of social rights.

Although his essay is relatively silent about the appropriate criteria by which to evaluate the reasonableness of citizenry demands, Marshall's invocation of the concept of "legitimate expectations" to define the content of social rights tracks the tenor of public debate about social issues. His insight is especially evident in recent government inquiries into the status of medicare in Canada. The federal government created the Commission on the Future of Health Care, and the Alberta government commissioned the Mazankowski Report (2001), largely in response to the fact that "Canadians express[ed] concerns about waiting lists and timely access to certain medical procedures" despite rising provincial expenditures (Romanow 2002, 4). The perception that lengthening waiting periods for non-elective surgery reflect a health care system in crisis reveals not only that citizens share expectations about how much time we should reasonably wait for medical procedures, but also that the current trend toward longer waiting lists illegitimately ignores this expectation.

Following Marshall's insights about the qualitative content of social rights, a central theme of this book is that the struggle over social citizenship amounts in large part to a struggle over public attitudes. The right-of-centre restructuring of the past two decades has been just as much about the state changing citizens' expectations as it has been about changing government budgets (Kline 1997, 349; Workman 1996, 15). From a neoliberal perspective, many Canadians demonstrate too little self-reliance and personal responsibility and have lost sight of the independence attainable from a strong commitment to labour markets and their families (Richards 1997, 144-45). As a result, some economic conservatives are concerned that citizens increasingly fail to recognize the limits and liability of government provision. Reorienting public attention to the value of a circumscribed state has, therefore, become a primary neoliberal objective, as we will see in the next chapter.

The question of legitimate citizen expectations also informs the revised framework for social citizenship that I propose in Chapters 7 and 8. My argument that caregiving should be built into the meaning of Canadian citizenship rests on the claim that successfully combining the aspirations and obligations associated with both caring *and* earning is a legitimate expectation among individual Canadians that ought to be officially recognized by the state. This theme is developed throughout the book by referencing a number of social factors – labour market transitions, declining real wages for men, and families' shifting organizational strategies – that highlight the pragmatic need for work-family balance, as well as social justice considerations – demands of social security, equality, and dignified community membership – that give legitimacy to the expectation.

3
The Celebrated Idiot:
The Obliged Citizen

I remember back six years ago, this Western life I chose.
And every day, the news would say some factory's going to close.
Well, I could have stayed to take the Dole, but I'm not one of
those.
I take nothing free, and that makes me an idiot, I suppose.
– Stan Rogers, "The Idiot"[1]

Legendary Canadian folksinger Stan Rogers foreshadowed the rise of
duty discourse in Canada with his song "The Idiot." His lyrics implore
"fine young fellows" from the East Coast, "who've been beaten to the
ground" by unemployment, to forgo "the government Dole [that] will
rot your soul" in order to embark on a westward odyssey. Rogers concedes that "western life's no paradise," but "it's better than lying down,"
he maintains, because it holds open the possibility of "self-respect," "a
steady cheque," and freedom in the dust-filled refineries of oil-rich
Alberta.

The Idiot that Rogers celebrates in his narrative has since become the
heroic citizen envisioned by many policy reformers in Canada, including Courchene (1994a) and Richards (1997). Both scholars draw extensively on social science evidence to argue that the structure of postwar,
social liberal income security is dysfunctional. In their view, it perpetuates poverty by inducing citizens' dependency on social transfers of the
kind that Rogers warns against. For instance, Richards (144) explains
about unemployment insurance (UI) that,

in 1971, Ottawa undertook major liberalization of the program. As workers and employers adjusted to the post-1971 rules, UI became increasingly inequitable and inefficient: inequitable because it obliged those

in stable industries and low-use regions to pay a permanent subsidy to those in seasonal industries and high-use regions, and inefficient because it unduly induced workers and employers to postpone strategies of moving into higher productivity sectors. Given the magnitude of these effects, the program gradually lost credibility among the majority of Canadians. Although the underlying market failures of adverse selection mean that governments can potentially improve both equity and efficiency by organizing universal social insurance against bouts of *unanticipated* unemployment, the Canadian system became an ongoing subsidy to bouts of *anticipated* unemployment.

Richards (1997, 144-45) supports this analysis with data showing that between 1971 and 1992 "repeat users became an increasingly important share of UI beneficiaries. The probability that a repeat user ... would initiate a claim in any year grew from approximately 50 per cent in 1972 to a peak of 80 per cent in the mid-1980s." Courchene (1994a, 36) corroborates this finding, reporting that, "in two New Brunswick counties, 100 per cent of two-earner households accessed UI at some time during 1992 and the ratio was well above 90 per cent for many other counties in Atlantic Canada." The trend that Richards and Courchene observe was not simply an East Coast issue. The "tourist industry in all provinces [became] geared to the existence of UI" (ibid.); workers would put in sufficient hours during the tourist season to draw on unemployment insurance during off-peak periods. On the West Coast, the concept of "fishing for stamps" signalled the same trend whereby some fishers would work only the time required to qualify for UI benefits. What these examples indicate, Courchene (ibid.) concludes, is the pervasiveness of "transfer dependency" in Canada. Invoking the concept of moral hazard, he urges that Canadians must "be prepared to contemplate that government largesse, at least as embodied in the current nature of our transfer envelope, is part of the problem rather than part of the solution" (43).

Courchene (1994a, 30) is careful not to blame individuals who fall subject to the welfare trap. The problem, he suggests, ultimately reflects a "system dysfunction" that does "not ... relat[e] to the character of individuals that may get caught in these transfer-dependency syndromes." The essence of the welfare trap, Courchene argues, is that the postwar welfare regime institutionalized incentives that have for decades interrupted the adjustment processes of the national economy, including inter-regional migration among the un(der)employed that Rogers urges in his song. This interference "was bound to serve to entrench and, in many cases, exacerbate the pre-existing degree of disparity [between citizens]" (29) since, "by and large, [benefit claimants] have acted *entirely rationally* in the face of a wholly inappropriate set of incentives" (30).

Courchene and Richards focus on three system failures inherent in postwar welfare programming. Overly generous benefits top their lists, with Richards (1997, 158) attributing much of the significant rise in welfare caseloads in Ontario during the 1980s and early 1990s to increasingly generous welfare benefits in the province. Tax rates for people leaving welfare in favour of employment represent a second failure (Courchene 1994a, 154; Richards 1997, 269). Courchene reports that "average tax rates in the transition from welfare to work frequently tend to be confiscatory by exceeding 100 per cent. This is especially true when one adds in the 'non-cash' components of welfare, such as free drugs, subsidized housing, and so on" (154). The third structural failure is the delivery of welfare benefits for children. Ontario data from 1992 revealed that employable single adults received $7,804 annually, whereas a single parent with one child received $15,772; with two children, $18,864; and with three children, $22,365. Comparable after-tax incomes from employment in the same year demanded annual salaries of $7,350, $18,425, $22,800, and $29,625 respectively. The market-income equivalencies were higher still among welfare recipients benefiting from subsidized housing, amounting to more than $32,000 for a single parent with three children. Courchene's point is that "few single parents on welfare can step into the workforce and command a $32,000 income. In effect, therefore, the so-called welfare trap is really due to the presence of children and how they are treated under welfare."

The system failures that allegedly induce transfer dependency mark the point of departure for Courchene's and Richards's alternative visions of social citizenship. Specifically, they ask us to reassess the nature and place of social duties in our conception of modern welfare regimes, particularly the duty to work. Marshall (1964, 118-19) recognized this duty in his initial research on social citizenship, calling upon each citizen to "put one's heart into one's job and work hard." But the commitment to a Protestant work ethic implicit in Marshall's position is elevated to a new status in the writings of Richards and Courchene (1994a, 326), who advocate the transition from welfare to workfare or "training-fare." According to Richards (1997, 257), "programs designed to aid the able-bodied unemployed should impose work and/or training conditions on the receipt of income transfers and should not accommodate long-term transfers to individuals if financial need is the only presenting problem." Given "what is known about social pathologies arising from long-term transfer dependence and the skills lost from extended unemployment," he argues that transfer programs which fail to institutionalize work requirements "pose serious disadvantages" (275). "Untied aid for the poor – such as long-term welfare – is a poisoned chalice. It has encouraged the poor to accept and even pursue extended periods without work, contrary to their own long-term interests, and it has damaged the stability of communities that have come to depend on transfers as the dominant source of income" (260).

Both Courchene and Richards assume that it is in the self-interest of unemployed citizens to be obliged to work or train as a condition of social assistance, particularly now that the domestic economy has evolved dramatically as a result of the diminution of resource-based industries and the simultaneous expansion of the information sector. This structural shift, they maintain, elevates the importance of human capital for personal security, including investments in education, training, and work experience. Courchene (1994a, 234) notes that a policy orientation organized around human capital was "not viewed as essential to our prosperity in an era when high school dropouts could earn 'middle-class' incomes in the forests, mines or energy sector." But the concept must now play a much more significant role, he argues, because burgeoning welfare caseloads include beneficiaries who are able to work, while the resource sector consistently produces fewer high-paying jobs for low-skilled labour. Courchene, therefore, recommends that Canada must move beyond a "resource-based mentality to a human-capital mentality" (ibid.). Top priority for social policy reform, he urges, should be to design "a set of programs geared to ensure that individual Canadians have both access and opportunity to enhance their skills and human capital" (240), since this capital will be necessary for citizens to function as "full participants in the Canadian and global societies" (339). Richards (1997, 264) articulates a similar position. He argues that "a crucial component [of future social policy] should be a political commitment to fund generous, lifetime training programs for all" and recommends that training "for nonprofessionals should be subsidized as generously as is university training for those pursuing professional careers."

The call for governments to expand lifelong learning programs signals that the alternative citizenship vision advanced by Richards and Courchene does not just entail spending reductions to mitigate policy incentives that allegedly erode employment incentives. Although cost-cutting factors importantly in their policy blueprint, they maintain that state "restructuring" is ultimately necessary to preserve social programs and prevent full "erosion" of the welfare system in this era of fiscal austerity (Courchene 1994b, 111; see also Richards 1997, 38). According to Courchene, extensive cuts in some areas must power reinvestment in other policy envelopes that have become more pressing with the knowledge economy revolution. Specifically, he thinks that major social programs such as "education/training, health, and income redistribution" must "transcend their traditional 'social focus'" so that they can be reorganized "in ways that contribute to both cohesion and competitiveness" (2001, 11). These programs "are major economic motors and export platforms in their own right," he insists. "If we fail to view them as both social and economic instruments, they will soon fail to deliver state-of-the art social programs" and in the process place at risk our country's social solidarity, as well as many citizens' abilities to thrive amidst the globalization and information revolution (ibid.).

The Rise of Duty Discourse

The invocation of the duty concept that motivates the human-capital policy reforms proposed by Courchene and Richards is consistent with scholarship from diverse political-ideological camps. It is, therefore, difficult to align their work definitively with a single analytic perspective. Rather than categorize Courchene or Richards at this stage, the objective in this chapter is simply to reveal the extent to which disparate schools of thought sympathize with the attention they accord to the concept of social obligation. Four schools of thought are reviewed in this chapter: neoliberalism, the third way, communitarianism, and social conservatism. The role that the concept of obligation plays in feminism is set aside at this point in favour of drawing extensively on feminist literatures in the next chapters with the intention of evaluating what is wrong and right about the various versions of duty discourse that have evolved in the last two decades.

Despite favouring opposite ends of the left/right political continuum, neoliberalism and third way versions of duty discourse align particularly closely with those of Courchene and Richards in that they prioritize employment duties. Both discourses critically target the social liberal preoccupation with state welfare and its vision of the citizen as a rights claimer. Communitarianism and social conservatism also share these two concerns about the social liberal paradigm, but they diverge from neoliberalism and the third way by articulating the critiques so as to challenge the liberal tendency to align autonomy with individualism at the expense of community order and tradition. The chapter concludes by linking the rise of duty discourse across political traditions with renewed interest in civic republicanism, which regards citizenship as a matter of participation just as much as status.

Neoliberalism

I use the terms "neoliberalism" and "economic conservatism" as synonyms. This political camp appropriates many classical liberal principles emphasizing freedom, market individualism, and laissez-faire government. The rhetorical significance assigned minimal government merits careful scrutiny, however, since neoliberal policy prescriptions regularly impose a *strong* state to mitigate market-blocking institutions or incentives (McBride and Shields 1997, 31), including unions, minimum wage legislation, and passive social assistance strategies. US thinkers Murray (1984, 1987) and Mead (1986, 1997a, 1997b) are among the school's most influential conceptual architects.

The commitment to free markets enshrined within neoliberalism stimulates structural changes affecting the family and other areas of social life that dramatically alter the relationship that economic conservatives hold with respect to tradition – "that very phenomenon," Giddens (1994, 2) notes, which conservatives "previously held most dear." One result is that modern economic conservatives are "conservative" in name only. The theoretically consistent neoliberal (although some are not!) advocates a philosophy that "is libertarian on moral as well as economic issues," offering support in favour of female employment (often in low-wage work), "sexual freedom," and "decriminalizing ... drugs" (Giddens 1999, 6).

Despite sharing the legacy of liberal theory, neoliberalism departs dramatically from its social liberal cousin. It downplays the role that social barriers, particularly systemic factors, play in explaining poverty and the marginalized status suffered by the less fortunate (for example, Mead 1997b, 48-50). Neoliberals, therefore, express considerable skepticism about the emphasis that Marshall and Rawls place on state welfare provision and social citizenship rights, casting doubt that they are necessary conditions to enable all citizens to take full advantage of their formal civil and political liberties.

In particular, economic conservatives charge that the predominantly class-based analysis implicit in the social liberal paradigm positions proponents to portray capitalism as "a system, not of equality, but of inequality" (Marshall 1964, 84). This depiction of markets, they suggest, inclines some social liberals to embrace a commitment to state welfare that expresses a fundamental hostility to market behaviour. This hostility not only risks overlooking the fact that generous social programs depend upon vibrant capitalist economies, but also obscures the potential for excessive redistribution to undermine economic efficiency, thereby limiting the welfare produced by labour and consumer markets, as well as the revenue available for public programming (Roche 1992, 82). In particular, research popularized by the Laffer curve reveals the possibility that reducing income tax rates that discourage the activity being taxed may lead individuals to work and earn more, with the result that government revenue actually increases.

Working from this analytic perspective, which shifts emphasis from state-based to market welfare generation, neoliberals argue that citizens have a social responsibility to insure themselves against social risks by developing the attributes and attitudes necessary to flourish and adapt in dynamic capitalist economies. The American scholar Mead (1986, 1997a, 1997b) is a particularly eloquent proponent of this view. He charges that social liberal welfare "programs that support the disadvantaged and unemployed have been permissive in character, not authoritative ... They have given benefits to their recipients but have set few requirements for how [recipients] ought to function in return" (1986, 1). Particularly harmful, Mead suggests, is that "government programs have given [the message] that hard work in available jobs is no longer required of Americans" (3). If employment conditions are disagreeable or remuneration too low, passive employment insurance and welfare programs institutionalize morally hazardous dynamics by relieving citizens of the responsibility to work for pay. The generosity of income assistance, coupled with the failure to obligate benefit recipients, does the disadvantaged a disservice, Mead maintains, by "undercutting" incentives to acquire "the competences [they] need to achieve status" and social belonging (12). The result, he concludes, is a population of social assistance recipients who are permitted to remain dependent on the largesse of the public sphere, rather than strive for self-sufficiency and self-respect, as does the Idiot in Rogers's song.

According to Mead (1986, 6), renewed interest in social obligations must extend well beyond a commitment to "paying taxes, obeying the law, or serving in the military." He argues that social order "also requires that people function well in areas of life that are not directly regulated," including the fulfillment of expectations that others hold about our roles as workers, neighbours, or strangers (ibid.). This expectation "requires not only self-discipline but *activity* and *competence*" (ibid.). Mead advocates a social order in which the population is encouraged to cultivate "those habits of mutual forbearance and reliability which we call civility," habits that are premised on "the capacities to learn, work, support one's family, and respect the rights of others" (ibid.). The attainment and exercise of these capacities constitute what Mead terms "a set of *social* obligations" that citizens incur as a condition of the privileges that accompany community membership (ibid.).

Mead's vision of social order, similar to the views of Courchene and Richards, has specific consequences for welfare policy design. He is sympathetic to the view that the remedy to transfer dependency involves revisiting the generosity of social assistance and redesigning social policy to minimize the disincentives to work imposed by confiscatory benefit clawback rates that accompany the move from welfare to work. But despite its significant cost, "expense is not the main objection to American 'welfare,'" he maintains (1997a, 202). "Far more significant are the effects these programs may have on the social functioning of the poor" (203). Thus, in some tension with more fervent antigovernment colleagues like Murray (1984), Mead (1997a, 222) argues that the fundamental change required is not so much to limit the cost of state welfare as it is to reorient the state to "complement welfare rights with obligations, both of them legally codified."

The concept of a reciprocal contract is at the core of this alternative vision of state welfarism, displacing entitlement as the leading maxim. "The idea," Mead (1997a, 221) explains, "is that the needy should receive aid, but only in return for some contribution to the society and not as an entitlement." Like Courchene and Richards, he surmises that the most important obligation to enforce is the duty to work. Once adults are "making an honest effort to support their families, that is enough to justify at least some assistance. Indeed, since work is the strongest social obligation, the mere fact of working establishes a strong presumptive claim to assistance" (Mead 1986, 244).

Mead's vision of welfare contractualism clearly departs dramatically from the American Express™ model of citizenship, which emphasizes the privileges of membership. He suggests that his vision is better captured by the Budweiser™ jingle "For all you do, this Bud's for you." As he explains, "Budweiser ads show workers, usually blue collar, struggling with some challenging task, then knocking off and socializing in the nearest tavern. The emphasis is on work effort and reward, and especially on the *connection between* them. The effort and the relaxation are *both* necessary, and neither would be meaningful without the other. Only men who have worked hard have earned the right to play, while work would be pointless unless rewards lay at the end of it" (1986, 243).

Anticipating critics, Mead (1986, 10) does not shy away from the charge that welfare contractualism and workfare are punitive, "nothing more than an elaborate way of 'blaming the victim.'" The charge is misguided, he argues, since proponents of social citizenship must recognize that transfer dependency has become pervasive partly because "social programs ... expect too little of their recipients, not too much" (ibid.). By obstructing the implementation of reciprocal expectations about how benefit recipients must function to earn public assistance, Mead contends that "exaggerated fears of victim-blaming" do not help the poor but become "a leading cause of dependency" (ibid.). From the economic conservative perspective, workfare is not so much a measure by which the state blames those who deviate from societal expectations as it is a means to "persuade them to *blame themselves*" (ibid.).

The theme of self-blame distinguishes Mead's work from that of Courchene, who we have seen claims that transfer dependency does not result principally from the character of the dependent, since policies produce hazardous incentives to which people respond rationally in their self-interest. By contrast, Mead argues that the theme of moral hazard must be supplemented with more politically controversial questions about the actual competence of long-term welfare recipients. Competence, in this context, connotes an individual's ability to make choices and behave in a manner that promotes her or his self-interest. According to Mead, this competence cannot be assumed among the poor; we cannot take for granted that it is simply social barriers that impede individuals' acting in their self-interest. This assumption is suspect, he argues, because extant welfare polices based on incentives that were designed to appeal to individual self-interest "have not shown much power to alter the behaviour of the poor" (Mead 1997b, 24). In particular, in the absence of legislated work obligations, he argues that "the effect of welfare incentives and disincentives on how many recipients work is remarkably small. This is hardly surprising, since not working and bearing children out of wedlock, the behaviours that do the most to precipitate the poverty of the working-aged, are themselves contrary to self-interest as most people understand it. They cause poverty or make it worse. If self-interest were a sufficient motivation, living in poverty and being on welfare should themselves motivate people to avoid or leave those conditions" (ibid.).

Implicit in this analysis is Mead's (1997b, 28) opposition to the assumption typical of economists like Courchene that all individuals, including the poor, "are rational maximizers who act to advance their own self-interest if not society's." No social science, he suggests, "that assumes an invariant, optimizing mentality can deal well with the self-defeating aspects of the poverty lifestyle. Understanding dysfunction requires positing a more complex psychology, where people fail to do what they themselves desire and thus fail to exhaust the potential of their environment" (ibid.).

The promotion of self-blame is not punitive, Mead maintains, since accepting personal responsibility is a necessary condition for genuine social inclusion and equality. Commenting on the United States, he argues that "true acceptance in ... society requires" that citizens face and fulfill social requirements, "such as work" (1986, 4). So long as welfare policy is passive, benefit recipients are "defined by their need and weakness, not their competence" (9). An adequate policy regime must, therefore, "require work as well as offer support ... if the recipients [are] to be integrated and not just subsidized" (14). In his view, only a reciprocal welfare contract combines social requirement with support "in a balance that approximates what the nondependent face outside of government. This treats the dependent like other citizens in ways essential to equality" (10). In contrast, postwar welfare "programs infringe equality in this sense as much as they serve it. They raise the income of the needy, but they also exempt them from work and other requirements that are just as necessary for belonging" (12).

For Mead (1986, 240), the social stigmatization and marginalization that accompany passive social assistance render work requirements for welfare recipients far less punitive and make salient their underlying "moral" motivation. Linking work requirements to social assistance is not simply an expression of the state's "self-interest" in managing expenditures, but is also a moral project designed "to ensure, for their own benefit and others', that recipients do in fact discharge the common obligations of citizenship" (ibid.).

The Third Way
The third way represents a strategy among social democrats, especially in liberal welfare regimes, to move beyond old-style social democracy in response to the political success enjoyed by neoliberals. Proponents favour an analytic perspective that rejects the left/right divide. They instead embrace some New Right critiques of the welfare policies that social democrats proudly nursed to life, while simultaneously charting an alternative to the neoliberal vision for policy renewal. Giddens (1999, 2000) is particularly influential in defining the third way, as is Esping-Andersen (2002) in more recent work.

Prominent among the right-of-centre critiques with which Giddens engages is concern about the passivity of postwar social policy. As he announces, neoliberals "are surely correct to worry about the number of people who live off state benefits" and to alert policy makers to the reality that "the higher the benefits the greater will be the chance of moral hazard, as well as fraud" (1999, 114-15). In contrast to Mead, however, Giddens does not go so far as to align transfer dependency with individual incompetence. Rather, he follows Courchene in emphasizing that transfer dependency is a system dysfunction unrelated to the character of benefit recipients: "It isn't so much that some forms of welfare provision create dependency cultures as that people take rational advantage of opportunities offered" (ibid.). According to Giddens, then, opponents of neoliberalism must countenance the fact that "benefits meant to counter unemployment ... can actually produce unemployment if they are actively used as a shelter from the labour market" (ibid.).

Heeding his own advice, Giddens (1999, 65) joins in the celebration of Rogers's Idiot. The "prime motto" of third way politics, he explains, is *"no rights without responsibilities."* Just as individualism and lifestyle diversity are expanding, so there should be a corresponding "extension of individual obligations" (ibid.) – "we need more actively to accept responsibilities for the consequences of what we do and the lifestyle habits we adopt" (37). While the theme of mutual obligation was present in old-style social democracy, Giddens suggests that it lay largely dormant within the shadows of postwar concerns about collective provision. This dormancy is no longer feasible, however, given emergent fears about the decline of civic-mindedness in recent decades. In his view, defenders of social provisioning can no longer assume that "social cohesion" can be "guaranteed by the top-down action of the state" (ibid.). Instead, he concludes that critics of neoliberal welfare must "find a new balance between individual and collective responsibilities" in their respective counterproposals (ibid.).

The judgment that top-down state action is inadequate signals Giddens's sympathy for the neoliberal charge that postwar welfare overextended the state's scope beyond legitimate boundaries. He concedes, "there is no doubt that in many countries the state, national and local, became too large and cumbersome" (2000, 57). Social science evidence, he argues, confirms that "it is no longer feasible, or desirable, to have very steeply graduated income tax of the sort that existed in many countries up to thirty or so years ago" (97). In place of the postwar welfare model, Giddens (1999, Chapter 4) urges instead that we should operationalize "the social investment state." The guideline for this state "is investment in *human capital* wherever possible, rather than the direct provision of economic maintenance" (Giddens 1999, 117). As it is for Mead, Courchene, and Richards, active labour policy is, thus, a top priority for Giddens. "Unemployment benefits," he claims, "should carry the obligation to look actively for work, and it is up to governments to ensure that welfare systems do not discourage active search" (65).

Despite appropriating these neoliberal insights, Giddens nonetheless retains a strong social liberal thrust in the third way, particularly in regard to the role he outlines for the state. The third way is fundamentally hostile to the idea of reducing state welfarism to a safety net of last resort that faithfully awaits the "trickle-down effects" of economic growth (Giddens 2000, 33). It favours instead "a welfare system that benefits most of the population" in order to "generate a common morality of citizenship" (1999, 108). This theme harkens back to the legacy of Marshall, who argued that social citizenship rights have the potential to foster social cohesion and a common sense of community membership among citizens. Where policy makers discount Marshall's insight, assigning welfare "only a negative connotation ... [that] is targeted largely at the poor," Giddens argues "the results are divisive," as is evident in the United States (ibid.).

Contra neoliberal thinking, Giddens is also adamant that human-capital investment and workfare alone do not capture the full scope of social provisioning for which the state must play an active role. Notwithstanding his assertion that "investment in education is an imperative of government today," he warns that "the idea that education can reduce inequalities in a direct way should be regarded with some scepticism. A great deal of comparative research, in the United States and Europe, demonstrates that education tends to reflect wider economic inequalities and these have to be tackled at the source" (Giddens 1999, 109-10). Similarly, he critiques neoliberal approaches to workfare on the grounds that "reducing benefits to force individuals into work pushes them into already crowded low-wage labour markets," whereas "involvement in the labour force, and not just in dead-end jobs, is plainly vital to attacking involuntary exclusion" (110).

In sum, the third way retains a robust role for welfare institutions, which ideally will "foste[r] psychological as well as economic benefits" (Giddens 1999, 117). State provision of income support and enforcement of employment obligations are, therefore, rarely seen to be sufficient.

Fighting poverty, according to Giddens (110-11), becomes part of a broader project of "community building" that "concentrate[s] upon the multiple problems individuals and families face, including job quality, health and child care, education and transport." Such a citizenship regime demands that "welfare expenditure remain at European rather than US levels," switching when necessary from passive to active income support measures to mitigate transfer dependency (122).

The social democratic distinctiveness of third way politics is manifest in comparison to the policy renewal urged by Courchene and Richards, who do not show a comparable commitment to a strong welfare state. Rather, they both argue for reinvestment in social policy primarily *because,* and only where, it "holds the key to regaining [Canada's] competitive edge" in the global economy (Courchene 1994b, 114; see also Courchene 1994a, 233; Richards 1997, 257-66). For Courchene and Richards, reinvestment in social programming appears to be conditionally valuable as a means to reinforce economic growth, rather than intrinsically important for fostering social inclusion or minimizing inequality. This perspective is consistent with organizing restructuring primarily around measures that promote workfare, which supplies low-skill labour for the growing service sector, and human-capital acquisition, which cultivates skilled labour to service expanding knowledge-based industries.

Communitarianism

Like "third way," the term "communitarian" has a relatively recent origin. Prominent scholars who align themselves with this political camp include Etzioni (1993, 1996) and Selbourne (1994). They share with Giddens the aspiration to push contemporary political debates about citizenship and social provisioning beyond the intellectual manacles of the left/right ideological divide (Etzioni 1996, 7; Selbourne 1994, 273). Yet, consistent with the New Right desire to substantially reduce state influence, communitarian policy prescriptions suggest strong support for the organization of welfare principally at small-scale community levels and by voluntary associations where possible. Devolution of responsibility is expected to improve upon the present reliance on federal and state/provincial government bureaucracies, which are allegedly more psychologically distant from citizens, not to mention more cumbersome and corrupt (for example, Etzioni 1996, 151-54).

While the term may be modern, communitarianism draws upon a long history that traces back to the ideas of Aristotle, through St. Augustine, Thomas Aquinas, Burke, and Hegel, and into work by contemporary scholars (though they resist the label) such as Sandel, MacIntyre, Walzer, and Taylor. The common denominator between these thinkers is a strong opposition to the assumptions about autonomy advanced by social liberalism, which aligns the concept with the entirely self-sufficient, rights-claiming individual. Communitarian sympathizers suggest this vision of autonomy goes astray because its atomistic predispositions obfuscate the social nature of individual agency. Liberal proponents are accordingly charged with failing to acknowledge and embrace adequately the social obligations to the community that are necessary to sustain and cultivate the interdependence that underpins individual autonomy. Thus, while social liberalism advances the politics of rights, communitarianism responds by urging renewed interest in the politics of the common good.

The reactionary character of contemporary communitarianism particularly laments the excesses of egoism and the evolution of the so-called Me generation that is allegedly less mindful of moral order, social tradition, and custom. It is "a corrective to excessive individualism," Etzioni (1996, 40) explains, one that does not pose a challenge to specific entitlements or to the idea of rights more generally so much as it seeks to restore balance to an era of overheated individualism. The objective is to thwart the advance of unconditional rights by reasserting "communitarian ideas and ideals [that] have been part of our intellectual heritage for a long time" (39), but which have been overshadowed by the rise of egoist aspirations. Selbourne (1994, 5) puts the need for this reassertion as follows:

> There is ... a now familiar form of ethical myopia. It is a product of – and further contribution to – the intellectual limitations of a mere politics of rights. Indeed, in corrupted liberal orders dominated by claims to dutiless right, demand-satisfaction and self-realisation through unimpeded freedom of action, a politics of rights amounts, in conditions of civic disaggregation and disorder, to little more than a politics of individual claims *against* the civic order and of duties owed by the latter *to* the individual. Missing consistently is a third term: the duties of the individual to himself and to fellow-members of the civic order to which he belongs.

The remedy that Etzioni (1996, 42) and other communitarians propose is "a *temporary* moratorium on the minting of *new* rights" in order to restore equilibrium between individual autonomy and obligation to communal order, rather than maximizing one over the other. For the communitarian, restoration of this equilibrium demands far more than simply enforcing the work duty that is of principal concern to neoliberals. It requires instead renewed commitment by every citizen to what Selbourne (1994, 222) terms "a general duty of care" for the ethical and practical condition of the civic order, which ultimately fosters individual well-being by determining the "degree of safety" that a citizen enjoys and nourishing "his capacity to realise his purposes as a moral being." Etzioni (1996, 43) illuminates the rationale for this general duty in less abstract terms. He argues that "sociological protection of a regimen of individual rights ... entails that the basic needs of the members of a community be served. This, in turn, requires that they will live up to their social responsibilities, from paying taxes to serving in neighborhood crime watches, from attending to their children to caring for their elders. No government alone can provide the needed services."

The general responsibility of care for the civic order "is the duty of a free citizen," Selbourne (1994, 222) maintains. This is not simply the freedom Rogers refers to in respect of the Idiot, who is free from the dole and empowered by the self-respect of a steady cheque. The freedom the communitarian is concerned with is much more foundational as it contemplates the societal conditions that are prerequisite for individual autonomy – conditions that theorists who assert the primacy of rights often ignore.

Social liberal protagonists of the primacy of rights, we have seen, value the kind of freedom by which citizens actively choose life-course paths from among a wide range of alternatives, arrive at self-selected definitions of personal goals, and discern for themselves what ideas and institutions command their allegiance. The communitarian point is that this autonomy is only possible within a cultural context that makes community members cognizant in a vivid way of the life-course options available, equips individuals with value systems by which to evaluate alternatives, and recognizes the enormous worth of freedom and individual diversity. A social fabric of this kind sustains and enables individuality. By contrast, a community rife with bigotry, intolerance, fear, or totalitarianism, or which simply devalues originality, innovation, and diversity in the name of efficiency and economic growth, risks undermining individual freedom. Thus, as Taylor (1992, 47) observes, "since the free individual can only maintain his identity within a society/culture of a certain kind, he has to be concerned about the shape of this society/culture as a whole." Primacy-of-rights theorists who neglect this fact in favour of atomistic tendencies therefore suffer what Taylor refers to as the "delusion of self-sufficiency which prevents them from seeing that the free individual, the bearer of rights, can only assume this identity thanks to his relationship to a developed liberal civilization; that there is an absurdity in placing this subject in a state of nature where he could never attain this identity and hence never create by contract a society which respects it. Rather, the free individual who affirms himself as such *already* has an obligation to complete, restore, or sustain the society within which this identity is possible" (49).

This communitarian critique is a bitter pill for the social liberal to swallow. It charges that social liberals like Marshall and Rawls insufficiently develop the social element of citizenship to fully contemplate the preconditions for liberty, despite the fact that they prioritize these conditions in their own work. The implications for one's understanding of what it means to be a full member of society are significant. Whereas the American Express™ model of citizenship emphasizes access to the range of community entitlements as the condition for full membership status, the communitarian adds that full membership demands specific activities on the part of the citizen. We are full members of a society only if we discharge sufficiently the social obligations necessary to sustain the community structures, values, and social attachments that make possible our liberty.

For the communitarian, the ideal would see citizens voluntarily perform the general duty of care they owe society. Etzioni (1996, 13), for instance, speaks of sustaining "voluntary compliance" through "normative means," such as "moral education," that will engender a shared "set of core values." As a result of such education, he believes that "the tension between one's preferences and one's social commitments [can] be reduced by increasing the realm of duties one affirms as moral responsibilities – not the realm of duties that are forcibly imposed but the realm of responsibilities one believes one should discharge and that one believes one is fairly called upon to assume" (12).

Selbourne (1994, 222-23), however, is not so sanguine about the likelihood that citizens will fulfill their obligations given the pervasiveness of ethical myopia. Accordingly, he affirms the neoliberal intention to employ the coercive power of the state to ensure individuals discharge their social obligations when necessary. As he puts it, the general responsibility of care and co-responsibility for social structures and practices "may, in the discretion of the civic order, be enforced by sanction in regard to the particular duties which it dictates" (ibid.).

Although members of the communitarian camp share a commitment to re-emphasize the value of community and social attachments, there is not agreement about which attachments and communities have particular value. Some, for instance, grapple with the legacy of oppression and hierarchy that pervaded traditional communities by proposing to rebuild small-scale institutions around social norms that embrace a greater commitment to equality. Etzioni's (1993, Chapter 3) lengthy discussion of the "communitarian family" captures this trend.

The family is an important institution to communitarians because they regard it as an incubator for the civility they fear is dissipating in public spaces. From this perspective, Etzioni (1993, 55) laments "the parenting deficit" that he believes is the cost of dual-earner families. While agreeing that women should have the same right as men to seek employment outside the home, in his view, this feminist concern is not the principal issue: "the issue is the dearth of parental involvement of both varieties: mothers and fathers" (ibid.).

> Few people who advocated equal rights for women favored a society in which sexual equality would mean a society in which all adults would act like men, who in the past were relatively inattentive to children. The new gender-equalized world was supposed to be a combination of all that was sound and ennobling in the traditional roles of women and men. Women were to be free to work any place they wanted, and men would be free to show emotion, care and domestic commitment. For children this was not supposed to mean, as it too often has, that they would be bereft of dedicated parenting. (63)

Etzioni's (1993, 64) communitarian reclamation of the family would, thus, return us "to a situation in which *committed parenting is an honorable vocation*" for both mothers and fathers. The alleged dishonour into which parenting has fallen in recent decades, and the resulting "widespread neglect of children" (63), he argues, contributes directly to the moral decay evident in "gang warfare ... drug abuse, [and] a poorly committed workforce" (69). "The time has come," he maintains, "for both parents to revalue children and for the community to support and recognize their efforts" (63). "We must acknowledge that as a matter of social policy ... we have made a mistake in assuming that strangers can be entrusted with the effective personality formation of infants and toddlers" (60). In place of non-parental child care services, Etzioni urges that communities should enable parents to take time away from paid employment to fulfill their shared responsibilities for childrearing. This includes new commitments to parental leave benefits (71-72), as well as revised labour usage strategies to allow "millions of parents to work at home" through telework, promote parents in dual-earner families to work "different shifts," or enable one parent to work "part-time" (70).

Some communitarians are less careful than Etzioni to acknowledge systems of inequality when they refer back to traditional families, neighbourhoods, and the church for inspiration in their attempt to diagnose the ailments of civil society and reassert communitarian ideals into contemporary politics. Even Etzioni's policy prescriptions regarding shared parental responsibility and part-time employment are very Pollyanna-ish about the gender division of labour, the disproportionate share of childrearing responsibility that women shoulder, and the extensive economic costs associated with part-time attachments to the labour market in which women predominate. In such instances, the boundaries between communitarianism and social conservatism blur considerably, so that the communitarian call for individuals to "act as responsible citizens often assumes women should fulfill their traditional roles" (Bussemaker and Voet 1998, 295).

Social Conservatism

Social conservatives are fervent advocates of moral traditions, defending the church and the idealized 1950s patriarchal family from the moral turpitude of feminism, homosexuality, sexual permissiveness, drugs, and consumerism. Like their neoliberal cousins, social conservatives employ rhetorical flourishes that laud small government. But this rhetoric again obscures the conservative's eagerness to legislate moral issues, provided that governments institutionalize "traditional," typically Christian, values that, among other things, are anti-gay and anti-abortion. In the United States, Berger and Berger (1983) and Gilder (1986, 1987) are notable social conservatives, as are their counterparts, Gairdner (1992) and, to a lesser extent, Smith (1997) in Canada.

Work by Giddens (1994, Chapter 1) reveals the inherent tension that exists between economic and social conservatives, since the former wish to unleash market forces that undermine traditional social structures, including practices that attract higher rates of female labour force participation. Despite this tension, the broader neoconservative political tent remains standing because both subgroups "share a desire to undermine their common enemy that is far more passionate than any desire to undermine one another" (Laycock 2002, 9). The common enemy is postwar welfarism. Social conservatives lend strong support to the neoliberal cause of shrinking the welfare state by charging that state welfare provision is instrumental in the demise of "traditional" families and Christian values because it obstructs citizens from fulfilling their private familial responsibilities. The disintegration of family discipline and sexual morality is in turn blamed for a number of social ills, including "juvenile delinquency and (increasingly) serious crime, drugs and alcoholism, suicide, a frenetic preoccupation with sexuality, mental disorders, and the appeal of fanatical cults" (Berger and Berger 1983, 160-61; see also Gilder 1987, 23-25).

Social conservatives allege that state welfare is culpable for attacking family values on several fronts. One is that welfare benefits ostensibly induce single mothers to marry the state rather than the fathers of their children. The shift to workfare exacerbates this problem by pushing unemployed mothers into the paid workforce and further eroding the need for a father or husband figure. Gilder (1987, 21) argues, for instance, that the "problem of hard-core poverty lies with violent and disruptive men and boys, not with unemployed women. Women already get most of the new jobs in America, particularly among the poor. *Female domination of work among the poor is the problem, not the solution.* Creating more employment and training for women – more advantages over their potential husbands – will only accelerate family decay."

A second social conservative indictment of welfare policy claims that the taxation required to fund state welfare imposes financial hardship on families that induces unnecessary female employment. In Canada, Gairdner (1992, 8) maintains that "high taxes are driving both spouses, willing or not, into the work force, consigning countless children to paid third-party care." Similarly, REAL Women of Canada (1999) suggests that the "real cause" behind the pressure for mothers with young children to seek paid employment "is that Canada has a punitive income tax structure." Absent from this line of criticism, however, is any acknowledgment of the evidence that shows Canada is below average among OECD countries in terms of the taxes that governments collect relative to GDP (Hale 2002, 20), or any recognition of the roads, national security, public utilities, medical insurance, etc., that citizens would need to pay for privately if they were not paid for publicly through taxes.

A third argument maintains that welfare state expansion has powered the increase in the numbers of social workers and other public sector "professionals" who prioritize their expertise above the practices of ordinary citizens and impose alien values on individuals and families (for example, Berger and Berger 1983, 210). The Bergers reject this use of "government power to influence or control behaviour within the family" (207). At issue, they insist, is "the extent to which parents are to be trusted to make decisions on the affairs of their children," regardless of their economic situation or educational status (212). "It is particularly odious, and empirically nonsensical," they contend, "to think that poorer and less educated parents are to be trusted less in those matters" (213). The Bergers, therefore, recommend the following "general maxim": "Trust parents over against experts; the burden of proof against individual parents should be very strong indeed before the opposite choice is made" to privilege professionals claiming to represent the best interests of children (ibid.).

The social conservative critique of state welfare essentially implores government to get out of the way of citizens assuming and fulfilling profound responsibilities to kin and other close relations. The patriarchal implications of this position for women are explicit. The Bergers (1983, 205), for instance, "hope" that many women "will come to understand that life is more than a career and that this 'more' is above all to be found in the family." REAL Women of Canada (2001) echo this sentiment, arguing that "women should have a genuine choice, financially and socially, to remain at home as full-time mothers, if they so choose, especially when their children are young."

This social conservative tenet is also evident in the work of Mead and Richards. Mead (1997a, 224) is explicit that child care assistance should be limited only to mothers who need to work to relieve the state of income-assistance responsibilities. Beyond this group, Mead is skeptical about the value of female labour force participation. In his view, joblessness today is due primarily to a growing labour force and job turnover. One overarching reason for the increasing pool of labour, Mead (1986, 71) claims, "is that more women and teenagers have been seeking jobs. While some members of these groups are responsible for their own households, many more of them, compared to adult men, are 'secondary' workers, from families where husbands, parents, or other members are already working ... While these workers clearly could use work, their joblessness cannot be viewed with the same seriousness as that of family heads, because they have other means of support."

Similarly, Richards (1997, 208) is emphatic that "family structure matters." He recommends that the state "discriminat[e]" fiscally in favour of two-parent families and expresses sympathy for the idealized patriarchal family of the 1950s (255-56). In his view, "commentators during the past generation have developed an important body of economic analysis that views traditional marriage as an efficient contract for the lengthy investment required for successful child rearing ... It is understood that each party will exploit his or her comparative advantage in order to maximize the joint interest in the success of the venture; the usual consequence (with many variants) is that mothers concentrate on child rearing, especially during the years of early child-hood, and fathers on earning income" (210-11).

While Richards (1997, 211) concedes that "feminists are right to lobby for a different distribution of benefits within marriage," he qualifies this concession by claiming it "is hard" to "measur[e] just how inegali-tarian marriages were in the past (and how egalitarian they are now)." With this qualification, Richards largely discounts extensive feminist literatures that are discussed in the next chapters. These literatures re-veal that welfare regimes premised on the "traditional" family have left women far more susceptible to poverty, violence, economic depend-ence, and social exclusion, and in the case of some poor, ethnic minor-ity, and immigrant women have marginalized them from their own domestic sphere.

In addition to supporting at-home motherhood, the social conserva-tive concern with familial duties also obliges fathers. This aspect of so-cial conservatism is principally a countercultural statement reasserting the importance of heterosexual men in response to the rise of single-motherhood, feminism, artificial insemination, and open lesbianism, which are interpreted as a societal declaration that heterosexual men are increasingly irrelevant (for example, Popenoe 1996). Gilder (1987, 21) articulates this position from a perspective that favours a strict division of gender roles: "We know, as much as we know anything, that only fathers can support families, reliably discipline teenage boys, and lift a community from poverty." He therefore advocates policies to supplement male wages, rather than displace them, in order to "reinforce the man's efforts as principal provider ... and ... keep him in his marriage" (24).

Popenoe (1996), by contrast, develops a more sophisticated position that would see fathers adapt to women's employment aspirations by cultivating what he describes as men's distinctly masculine capacity to nurture in addition to their aptitude for economic provision. For Popenoe, heterosexual men must cultivate their nurturing side in order to reclaim their preindustrial status as primary child-rearers, especially of older children. He contends that the involved father's contribution is irreplaceable when it comes to fostering intellectual achievement, em-pathy, and psychological well-being among children.

Hail the Modern Civic Republican

The emergence of duty discourses across disparate political traditions signals the revival of the active citizen, one who does not simply pursue self-selected goals, but who contributes to the definition and well-being of the communities in which she or he is a member. Whereas the social liberal model focuses on equal status, the citizenship vision that motivates the celebration of Rogers's Idiot is one conceptualized in terms of participation. This vision has strong roots in the tradition of civic republicanism articulated by Aristotle, Machiavelli, Rousseau, and Tocqueville, and has since been revised by scholars like Oldfield (1990).

For the civic republican, community is a much narrower concept than that accepted by the social liberal. It depends not so much on formal organization of institutions as it does on the sense of belonging and commitment that individuals share in regard to one another. Community, in this view, is something that must be generated; it exists, as Oldfield (1998, 89) puts it, only "wherever there are individuals who take the practice of citizenship seriously." This understanding of community implies a rigorous test of full membership in society. In effect, failure to engage with the duties and practices of citizenship signals that one is not acting as a full member or citizen, regardless of one's place of origin or passport.

The ethical impetus for civic republicanism traces back to an idyllic reinterpretation of Greek city-states in which the native-born male citizen is not simply a subject of a political community; he is involved politically, collaborating with fellow citizens to determine mutually their common destiny. Aristotle introduced this idea to us, arguing for a system of values in which regular political participation is an intrinsic good – an expression of freedom – and not simply instrumentally valuable for its contribution to other ends. Anticipating the anti-atomistic sentiments of contemporary communitarians, Aristotle portrays the citizen as a social animal who is not self-sufficient outside the boundaries of a polis. To the extent that one is dependent on social cooperation for mutual advantage and the defence of individual liberty, he implies that the citizen realizes a more robust freedom if he contributes to shaping society and the collective identity. Thus, Oldfield (1998, 79) maintains that, rather than constraining individual autonomy, the Aristotelian legacy teaches that institutional forces that motivate individuals to engage in the practice of citizenship "enable them to reach a degree of moral and political autonomy which a rights-based account cannot vouchsafe" (see also Taylor 1992).

Some contemporary civic republicans share with social liberalism an understanding of social citizenship that includes the collective provision of the socioeconomic conditions necessary for full community participation. For instance, Oldfield (1998, 79) argues, "civic republicanism recognizes that, unsupported, individuals cannot be expected to engage in the practice [of citizenship]." He continues:

> Resources can be seen as enabling or empowering individuals to be active agents in this world. For activity of any kind, including that involved in the practice of citizenship, people need certain resources. Some of these have to do with what liberal individualism identifies as civil, political and legal rights. Others have to do with economic and social resources. Without health, education, and a reasonable income, for instance, individuals do not have the capacity to be effective agents in the world, and the possibilities of a practice of citizenship are thus foreclosed. Such rights and resources have to be secured for citizens, for citizenship is an egalitarian practice. (86-87)

But the civic republican is not satisfied with an understanding of social citizenship that stops with the provision of socioeconomic resources and opportunities. For Oldfield (1998, 87), these are "not sufficient for the practice of citizenship." Individuals must also have sufficient self-motivation to participate. "What is further required," he explains, "is that a particular attitude of mind be encouraged, an attitude which not only prompts individuals to recognize what their duties are as citizens, but which motivates them to perform them as well. The problem to be overcome is that of the 'free-rider'" (ibid.). The only solution, he argues, is for the community to inculcate within its members what Tocqueville famously termed "habits of the heart" by which citizens internalize a covenant to accept co-responsibility for the common good.

Given its intellectual roots – Aristotle, Machiavelli, and Rousseau – the civic republican tradition is replete with gendered assumptions. All three thinkers align citizenship with masculinity, celebrating the political sphere as the realm of freedom, and they are wary about encumbrances present in private spaces that threaten public participation, including financial need and domestic responsibilities (Bussemaker and Voet 1998, 285). This theme remains evident in the work of Oldfield (1998, 81), who argues that "the practice of citizenship means that much more of one's life is lived publicly than is the case in the modern world. It is not that one has no private life; it is rather that to be a citizen is to be politically active, and political activity takes place in the public domain."

The single-mindedness of republicanism as to the venue for citizenship activity underscores the severity of this political tradition. Citizens are implored to be mindful of "important tasks which have to do with the very sustaining of their identity" and which do not permit "a re-laxed and private leisure" (Oldfield 1998, 79). But as Walzer (1991) notes, the severity of this vision is out of step with what is realistic for most people today. Not only does the scale of the modern democratic state mean that political power is not fully in the hands of the vast majority of citizens outside of electoral campaigns, but formal politics also rarely attract the full attention of citizens, since the need to make a living and tend to family and other intimate relations poses serious time constraints.

In response, we can understand the duty discourses of the four political camps considered in this chapter as offering a corrective to civic republican single-mindedness without relinquishing the expectation that citizenship indeed demands individual contribution to the common good. Neoliberalism and the third way elevate employment to the status of a vital citizenship practice and obligation. These traditions contend that individuals make a significant contribution to society by taking reasonable efforts to financially provide for themselves and their dependants and by paying taxes so that the collective can support the well-being of the less fortunate. In addition, although paid work begins as a necessity, neoliberal and third way proponents recognize that employment often assumes its own value, which individuals express through their commitment to career, pride in work completed, and ca-maraderie among co-workers.

Conversely, duty discourses in communitarianism and social conservatism identify the sphere of the family as an important locus for citizenry activity. The family, in these traditions, is seen as a seedbed for the civic virtues that their proponents warn are dissipating in modernity. It is also home to fundamental social attachments to kin and other cherished relations that become foundational for any sense of social belonging.

Both sets of improvements upon classical interpretations of civic republicanism have enormous value. I explore this value in more detail in the next chapter.

4

The Idiot's Acumen

There is much to celebrate and much to remain cautious about in re-obliging citizens to address the permissiveness of social liberal conceptions of citizenship. The question "What's right?" about this political-cultural trend is the principal concern in this chapter. The question "What's wrong?" about the obliged citizen envisioned by neoliberals, the third way, communitarians, and social conservatives is the subject of Chapters 5 and 6.

The normative framework within which I evaluate the various critiques of the American Express™ citizenship model is a feminist one. In this chapter I draw principally on the feminist literature spawned by Gilligan's (1982) original work on the ethic of care. Her empirical research in moral development challenged dominant traditions in social science, law, and philosophy, showing that these disciplines typically prioritize a single moral orientation that focuses on questions of justice from the perspective of liberal individualism. Just as we saw that Rawls's (1971) original position is premised on the assumption of mutual disinterest, so Gilligan (1995, 121) argues that "the voice that set the dominant key in psychology, in political theory, in law and in ethics, was keyed to separation: the separate self, the individual acting alone, the possessor of natural rights, the autonomous moral agent." This focus on separation, she maintains, distorts the role of relationships in human experience because it fails to account for connection other than by portraying it as a potential impediment to autonomy or an instance of self-sacrifice. The distortion, in turn, renders suspect the adequacy of contemporary moral, legal, and political practices that embody classical liberal commitments to rights and liberty insofar as they are premised on this atomistic approach.

The singular focus on separation in what Gilligan terms the ethic of justice risks ignoring the reality that connection with others is often "experienced as a source of comfort and pleasure, and a protection against isolation" (Gilligan 1987, 32). The result, she contends, is that many liberal approaches to scholarship fail to recognize that the justice framework is not the only moral orientation from which men and, especially, women deliberate when engaged in moral decision making. Gilligan finds that a second orientation, what she refers to as the ethic of care, is also pervasive. The second orientation is grounded on the assumption that relatedness is more fundamental than separation. It encourages individuals to recognize that connections with others imply mutual responsibilities and an imperative to respond actively to the needs of others, while it also cautions against uniform application of abstract principles in favour of remaining sensitive to contextual variation when deliberating morally.

The empirical findings provided by Gilligan suggest that a majority of North Americans invoke such care considerations when deliberating about moral issues, in addition to employing the justice framework on which research traditionally focused. As she explains: "Since everyone is vulnerable both to oppression and to abandonment, two moral visions – one of justice and one of care – recur in human experience. The moral injunctions, not to act unfairly toward others, and not to turn away from someone in need, capture these different concerns" (Gilligan 1987, 20).

While a majority raise both care and justice considerations during moral deliberation, Gilligan's work also indicates that roughly two-thirds of men and women tend to focus predominantly on the issues that are salient from a single perspective. Her studies reveal significant sex differences in the frequency with which individuals focus on either the care or the justice orientation (Gilligan 1987, 25). Invariably, men who focus are found to prioritize justice considerations, while women who focus divide roughly equally between the care and justice perspectives. Although a care focus is by no means characteristic of all women, the finding that this focus is almost exclusively a female phenomenon prompted a popular-culture mischaracterization of Gilligan's work in which the care ethic is identified exclusively with women's morality. This cultural (mis)interpretation is problematic since it risks reinforcing role specialization along gender lines on the assumption that women are "naturally" and ethically more inclined to care, nurture, and respond to the needs of others.

In contrast to popular-cultural misinterpretations, Gilligan's research also motivated numerous feminist scholars to investigate further what is implied by the ethic of care for moral and political theory, as well as to determine more clearly its relationship to the alternative justice perspective. The near consensus in the literature now is that both justice and care paradigms are extremely valuable for moral deliberation (see Held 1995). The question outstanding is how best to integrate the distinct and often competing interpretations of a moral problem that the two perspectives yield. As Held explains, "what remains to be worked out ... is how justice and care and their related concerns fit together. How does the framework that structures justice, equality, rights, and liberty mesh with the network that delineates care, relatedness, and trust?" (128). A variety of scholars have responded to this question, offering alternative ways to synthesize the focus on rights inherent in the justice paradigm with the attention to mutual responsibility urged by the care ethic's concern with connection (Card 1988; Dillon 1992; Friedman 1993; Kymlicka 2002, Chapter 9; Lister 1997a; Narayan 1995; Okin 1989; Tronto 1993). The resulting literature is rich with insights about the value of renewed political interest in social obligations, as well as the adequacy of the disparate visions of the obliged citizen that were considered in the previous chapter.

The Interdependent Citizen

The feminist debates motivated by Gilligan confirm the need to revisit and transcend the social liberal paradigm in order to address the risk of dutiless rights. The care orientation depicts moral problems in terms of conflicting responsibilities rather than competing entitlements. It also affirms the value that contemporary duty discourses ascribe to the active citizen. Responsibility, according to the ethic of care, signals the need for response, "an extension rather than a limitation of action" (Gilligan 1982, 38). Whereas negative rights that dominate the liberal ethic of justice primarily impose restraints on aggression, responsibility in the care paradigm demands an active response to the needs of others, one that requires we *do* what others are counting on.

Beyond the general support this literature lends to duty discourses, it also applauds the communitarian and social conservative invocation of the language of care to describe some citizenry obligations and aspirations. A moral paradigm that integrates an adequate appreciation for the reality of human connection treats caregiving as a fundamental moral activity and, therefore, prescribes care as a necessary element of many citizenry practices. Care is often necessary, Held (1995, 131) suggests, since "when, in society, individuals treat each other with only the respect that justice requires, the social fabric of trust and concern can be missing or disappearing."

But care duties are not strictly a citizenry issue because they underscore the trust and mutual respect that civic-mindedness demands in public spaces. As with communitarians and social conservatives, who identify the sphere of the family as an important locus for citizenry activity, so the care ethic challenges the public/private divide that informs civic republican and liberal citizenship traditions. Care provision in the private sphere of home and family emerges as a valuable citizenship contribution because, as Tronto (1993, 162) observes, "it is a part of the human condition that our autonomy occurs only after a long period of dependence, and that in many regards, we remain dependent upon others throughout our lives." The result is that caregiving in domestic spaces is an under-recognized issue for the socially engaged citizen. In some life-course periods, one is enabled to participate publicly just by virtue of the care one receives from parents, kin, or close relations; on other occasions, the engaged citizen facilitates the participation of others through his or her own care work. The care ethic literature thus affirms the communitarian depiction of the family as a foundational social institution with which scholars of citizenship must engage, particularly when it is accompanied by Etzioni's call to transform the gender relations that historically characterized this social domain. The objective is to acknowledge the moral values implicit in the caring practices and family ties on which human life depends so as to determine how social infrastructure can better support citizens in their efforts to embrace and abide by these values (Held 1995, 132).

At the conceptual level, this objective demands that we rethink the social liberal vision of autonomy. The tendency to align autonomous agency with the unencumbered pursuit of personal projects risks equating autonomy with the abandonment of care responsibilities that exist within the domestic sphere. One can only approximate a relationally unencumbered status if one exploits subordinate groups by transferring care obligations for dependants to others who, as a consequence, compromise their own autonomy by disproportionately shouldering care labour. If we reject this exploitation to minimize inequalities across sex, race, and class lines, the assumptions about autonomy that inform social liberalism must be refined so that autonomy is not thought to be achieved at the expense of fulfilling care duties.

Work by Kymlicka (2002, Chapter 9) regarding the relationship between the ethics of care and justice has been particularly insightful about this point. He observes that the Rawlsian concern to codify moral principles for citizens contributes significantly to preserving what he refers to as the "predictability" required for "meaningful autonomy" (416).

Moral principles provide guidelines by which citizens can distinguish in advance circumstances in which they owe responses to others from situations in which the subjective frustrations of others are a matter for which the persons in need are personally accountable as agents who are responsible for the consequences of their own actions. This advance knowledge is important, Kymlicka argues, because,

> if our aim is to ensure that the free pursuit of one's projects is not entirely submerged by the requirements of ethical caring, then we do not simply need limits on our moral responsibilities, we also need *predictable* limits. We need to know *in advance* what we can rely on, and what we are responsible for, if we are to make long-term plans. It is not much good being told at the last minute that no one needs your moral help today, and that you are free to take a moral holiday, as it were. We can only take advantage of holidays if we can plan them, and that requires that we can determine *now* which interests we will be held responsible for *later.* (415)

While the original position may help to identify principles of justice that retain the predictability necessary for autonomy in interactions between mentally competent, able-bodied adults, Rawls's thought experiment sidesteps a more significant challenge posed by the unpredictable needs and demands of dependants. Children, for instance, cannot be expected to demonstrate the same level of personal responsibility for their own needs and preferences, or to engage in relations of reciprocity whereby they show equal concern for preserving and fostering the autonomy of persons from whom they receive care (Kymlicka 2002, 415, 418). Similarly, the needs of the sick, elderly, or otherwise dependent are often not a matter over which they have control or that they can manage independently, and, again, this undermines their capacity to show reciprocal concern not to limit the autonomy of their care providers.

Kymlicka thus acknowledges that the mutually disinterested status typically assigned agents in liberal theory largely discounts the constraints on predictability that domestic care for dependants can impose. Summarizing findings from decades of feminist literature, he reports that much liberal theory either ignores "the nurturing of children and caring for dependents," assumes this work will "be somehow 'naturally' dealt with in the family, which ... fall[s] outside of the scope of a theory of justice" (2002, 417), or presumes "that some people (women) will 'naturally' desire to care for others, as part of their plan of life, so that the work of caring for dependents is not something that imposes moral obligations on all persons" (418).

If we are to shed the vestiges of patriarchy that underpin these misguided assumptions, there are significant consequences for liberal presumptions about autonomy. As Kymlicka (2002, 419) puts it: "Once people are responsible for attending to the (unpredictable) demands of dependents, they are no longer capable of guaranteeing their own predictability" to the degree presumed in the original position. If this predictability cannot be guaranteed, questions arise as to whether we can "meet our responsibilities for dependent others without giving up the more robust picture of autonomy" that underpins Rawlsian theory and the social institutions it informs (420). "Justice theorists," he concludes, "have constructed impressive edifices by refining traditional notions of fairness and responsibility. However, by continuing the centuries-old neglect of the basic issues of child-rearing and care for dependents, these intellectual achievements are resting on unexamined and perilously shaky ground. Any adequate theory of sexual equality must confront these issues, and the traditional concepts of discrimination and privacy that have hidden them from view" (ibid.).

The foundation needed to restore some stability to the shaky ground that Kymlicka diagnoses can be found partly in the strong opposition that communitarians and, to a lesser extent, social conservatives express in regard to the atomistic assumptions about autonomy that pervade social liberalism. By rejecting separation as the foundational assumption about human experience, the ethic of care develops the communitarian attentiveness to the social nature of individual autonomy and, especially, the interdependence that is its prerequisite. The liberal preoccupation with a separate self for whom autonomy is allegedly self-generated is rejected on grounds that this vision is intrinsically problematic morally. It signals a lack of awareness of the human interaction and mutual reliance in which people must be immersed before they can develop the moral capacities necessary to interpret events and respond to the recognition of responsibility for one another that interrelatedness implies. As Baier (1985, 84) explains, a morally autonomous agent is perhaps "best seen as one who was long enough dependent upon other persons to acquire the essential arts of personhood." Every autonomous individual experiences

> a childhood in which a cultural heritage is transmitted, ready for adolescent rejection and adult discriminating selection and contribution ... Persons are essentially successors, heirs to other persons who

formed and cared for them, and their personality is revealed both in their relations to others and in their response to their own recognized genesis. Not only does each earlier phase causally influence each later phase, as in all enduring things, not only is there growth, maturation, and aging, as in all living things, but in persons each later phase is a *response* to earlier phases, caused not only by them but by some sort of partial representation of them and their historical causal relationships. (85)

This rich appreciation for the fact that autonomy is only possible as a result of the social relations and infrastructure that nourish it parallels the communitarian sympathies that Taylor (1992) manifests in his diagnosis that liberal theorists who accord primacy to rights suffer the delusion of individual self-sufficiency. Taylor has subsequently developed his critique by further embracing the sort of analysis that Baier advances. He captures the fundamental connection between care relationships and human agency with his recognition that the genesis of personal autonomy is not monological, something we each achieve on our own, but *"dialogical"* (Taylor 1994, 32). "We become full human agents," he argues, "capable of understanding ourselves, and defining our identity, through our acquisition of rich human languages of expression" (ibid.). Taylor uses the term "language" in a broad sense, referring not only to the words we speak, but also to "other modes of expression," such as "the 'languages' of art, of gesture, of love, and the like" (ibid.). Other formative vocabularies include fluency in societal expectations, communal depictions of history, and the range of possible life paths articulated by cultural contexts. Taylor observes that "we learn these modes of expression through exchanges with others. People do not acquire the languages needed for self-definition on their own. Rather, we are introduced to them through interaction with others who matter to us – what George Herbert Mead called 'significant others'" (ibid.).

Social conservatives who view the family as a primary socializing and morality-engendering institution in modern society also implicitly subscribe to the dialogical thesis. For instance, like Taylor, social conservative sociologists Berger and Berger (1983, 165) build on Mead's recognition of the contributions of significant others to the genesis of the self. "The family," they claim, "is the necessary social context for the emergence of the autonomous individuals who are the empirical foundation of political democracy" (172). Infancy and early childhood serve "as the matrix ... for everything the particular individual will be and think in later life. In these early years ... both personality (or identity) and consciousness are formed" (150). For the Bergers, parents contribute most significantly to the moral norms that individuals internalize as children, representing "the strongest possible models for the performance of adult roles. Even when the child, in the process of growing up, struggles with and against these models, they are indispensable in serving as points of orientation" (162).

The constitutive role that others play in the formation and evolution of self-understanding, and the autonomous action this understanding permits, is most evident while we are infants, children, and youths. This role is so obvious in the early years that most thinkers who are committed to the alignment of autonomy and individualism are likely to concede willingly, as Rawls (1971) in fact does in Chapter 8 of *A Theory of Justice,* that our identities and personal projects are shaped significantly by the influence of people who nurture us (or fail to do so) during childhood. Despite granting this point, though, persons with individualist inclinations about autonomy may nonetheless reject the dialogical character as a suitable starting point to develop an account of human agency.

For instance, Tronto (1993, 163) observes that many political theorists who work in the tradition of Smith and Rousseau regard the life-course transition from stronger dependence toward greater individuation as a fact that merits particular attention in theories of agency. In this tradition, the important influence of others during early childhood development does not negate the fact that we should strive to define ourselves on our own terms as much as possible because dependent people risk losing "the ability to make judgements for themselves, and end up at the mercy of others on whom they are dependent" (ibid.). Accordingly, recognition of the dialogical character of childhood implies that we should try to arrive at some understanding of, and, therefore, some control over, the influence that immediate family members and others hold over us while we are maturing. Furthermore, although we may wish to acknowledge the contributions that others make to the formation of self-understanding, it is not obvious that we should seek similar relationships of dependence as adults that may mean we lose control over external influences. Rather, for persons inclined to align agency with individualism, it may appear that we achieve autonomy only when we are free to think, choose, and act independently for ourselves unconstrained by the attitudes, opinions, and actions of others. Therefore, the most appropriate starting point for analyses of human agency, the argument continues, is the recognition that autonomous agents are first and foremost sufficiently independent from the undue influence that others can impose.

While this critique raises legitimate worries about the proposal to revisit the link between autonomy and individualism, insights about agency advanced by feminists working in the tradition of Gilligan, as well as some communitarians and social conservatives, show that the above reasoning is wrong for two reasons. To begin with, the dialogical character of the human condition is not simply a fact about the genesis of our identities (Taylor 1994, 32). Our sense of self, our understanding of where we are coming from and, perhaps more importantly, where we are going, is never permanently fixed or stagnant. Rather, the feminist scholar Code (1987, 363) explains that we have a propensity to be influenced by others throughout our lives, which leaves us always "open to the effects of an interdependence." The Bergers (1983, 165) add that "significant relationships are important throughout life for the maintenance of identity and meaning." On one hand, persons continually reinterpret and respond to past experiences. We remain in dialogue with, and often struggle against, the views expressed by people who have been significant in our lives. Taylor (1994, 33) comments that, "even after we outgrow some of these [significant] others – our parents, for instance – and they disappear from our lives, the conversation with them continues within us as long as we live." On the other hand, our patterns of interaction also change. Over time we establish new relationships that may illuminate a range of values and interests that were not salient during earlier periods. By broadening our horizons, new relationships encourage the reassessment of our histories, motivations, and goals. Thus, as Baier (1985, 85) explains, "responses to dependency, and to changing degrees of it, to change of person on whom to depend, define our emotional life, form and display personality."

The individualist's concern that the dialogical thesis fails to appreciate the risks for autonomy which result from the lack of control we have over the influence that other persons wield on our identities is also misplaced. It is important to distinguish between the claim that our sense of self is shaped through interactions with others and the claim that others construct our identities for us. In accounting for human experience, the dialogical thesis does not depict the self as formed only by the ideas, values, and actions of others. The point is that the self is *in dialogue* with these things. Baier (1985, 85) and the Bergers (1983, 162) concur that the transmission during childhood of a cultural heritage infused with values and a range of sanctioned and proscribed life paths is subject to adolescent skepticism and adult reformulation.

Once equipped with some set of languages of expression and arts of personhood, we enter into a life of exchanges with other persons. We bring to these engagements our unique personality, creativity, and intellectual inclinations, characteristics that first develop largely in response to the way our natural talents were cultivated and our weaknesses emerged during early dependence. Sometimes exchanges result in our criticizing the values that others hold; on other occasions we may internalize them. Whatever the result, the dialogical thesis acknowledges that we normally contribute significantly to the exchange (Code 1987, 363).

Accepting as foundational the dialogical character of the human condition, therefore, does not impute a lack of control, loss of autonomy, or absence of individuality to the self "so long as 'individuality' is not equated with 'individualism'" (Code 1987, 361). The assumption implicit in the unencumbered self – that we act autonomously only when our reasons for action originate from a self-defined sense of what matters in life – is intuitively attractive. But the relational disconnection and inattention to unpredictable care responsibilities implicit in the original position discount how we achieve this self-definition. By contrast, some social conservatives, feminists, and communitarians illuminate how our sense of self is as much dependent on social and environmental relationships as it is upon what might be termed our own nature. The dialogical thesis, therefore, does not deny anything "of personal uniqueness, creativity, expressiveness and self-awareness" (ibid.). Rather, as Code observes, the thesis shows how "all of these grow out of interdependence, and continually turn back to it for affirmation and continuation" (ibid.).

In sum, the dialogical thesis appropriately transcends the liberal dualism that pits self-determination against interconnectedness. In place of mutually disinterested, relationally unencumbered actors who discount the unpredictable care demands of dependants, the thesis instead envisions individuals as persons-in-relations who move along a continuum of separation and connection that tracks life-course changes. As Held (1995, 132) has argued, "this relational view is the better view of human beings, of persons engaged in developing human morality. We can decide to treat persons as individuals, to be the bearers of rights, for the sake of constructing just political and other institutions. But we should not forget the reality and the morality this view obscures. Persons *are* relational and interdependent. We can and should value autonomy, but it must be developed and sustained within a framework of relations of trust."

Employment and Emancipation

The support the Gilligan-initiated literature lends to the communitarian critique of social liberal atomism is not unqualified, however. While human connection is indeed often experienced as a source of comfort and protection against isolation, a feminist care ethic does not deny that interrelatedness can also pose an obstacle to autonomy, just as the justice perspective warns. Feminists have long lamented the inequalities of power implicit in expectations of feminine selflessness and self-sacrifice that inform the gender distribution of care. Lister (1997a, 109) accordingly urges caution about "uncritical usage of the language of interdependence." If we are too sanguine about this theme, she warns, we risk ignoring that "the unequal power relationship that underpins [some] women's economic dependence on men means that the interdependence of which the dependence is a part is skewed in men's favour. It is not surprising, therefore, that the other element of the equation – men's dependence on women for care and servicing, which facilitates their own independence as citizens and workers – is conveniently obscured" (ibid.).

The short end of the interdependence stick has been a primary object of criticism for feminists since the movement's second wave. Friedan's (1963) *Feminine Mystique* prompted a new level of concern in North America about the social and economic marginalization suffered by many women as a result of their primary responsibility for domestic and care work in the family. The ensuing identification of employment as a necessary condition for full social membership for women converges unmistakably with neoliberal and third way proponents who regard paid work as a principal badge of social citizenship. Even the paternalism that runs throughout the policy prescriptions of Mead, Courchene, and Richards finds a feminist analogue. Just as the former invoke state levers to push citizens into employment for their own good, so the women's movement engaged in "consciousness raising" in the 1970s as part of a political strategy to lobby for pay and employment equity as well as child care in order to facilitate women's employment.

Feminist analyses that embrace what Gilligan (1987, 32) terms an "essential ambivalence" to human connection by acknowledging that care is a site of both immense satisfaction and deep discrimination share with neoliberalism and the third way a strong employment-based critique of postwar welfare. Many feminists, for instance, charge the welfare state with enshrining policy norms that obstructed women's access to employment. In Canada, the federal government's decision to withdraw wartime funding for child care is perhaps the most blatant example.

The Second World War resulted in a labour shortage to which Prime Minister Mackenzie King responded with the Dominion-Provincial Wartime Day Nurseries Agreements[1] as part of a plan to attract women to fill industrial positions left vacant by men who joined the armed forces. The agreements committed the federal government to share with provinces the costs of creating child care centres for mothers working in war-related industries and later extended this benefit to working mothers more generally. While only Quebec and Ontario made use of the federal funding, the agreements facilitated a significant transfer of responsibility for childrearing between family and state during the war years within these provinces. The transfer was short-lived, however. As industry's need for the supplementary labour of women subsided following 1945, Ottawa withdrew its financial support for child care, and many of the centres created in Ontario and Quebec closed (Baker 1995, 199; Childcare Resource and Research Unit 2000, 35, 44).

The elimination of federal child care funding illustrated the dominant societal expectation that the "good" mother would serve as a homemaker outside the paid labour market, particularly during her children's formative years. This cultural ideal marked a cornerstone of postwar social citizenship that partitioned the full range of human needs and aspirations, especially those related to reproduction and nurturing, labour market activity, as well as civic participation. Cross-national feminist analyses have found that the postwar political commitment to foster high and stable levels of employment was only made in respect of able-bodied men and never engaged the employment needs or aspirations of women in liberal welfare regimes (for example, O'Connor, Orloff, and Shaver 1999). Instead, women in private homes were expected to accommodate most of the vital day-to-day needs of children, the elderly, the sick, and persons with disabilities. As "mothers of the nation," their care labour (as well as that provided by poorly paid domestic help) did not simply raise the next generation of citizens. It also absolved many men, the state, and the marketplace of the largest share of daily welfare provision, making possible a dramatically different and elevated citizenship status for racially and economically privileged males. Unencumbered by many relational obligations of care and nurturing, financially secure men were positioned to approximate the liberating vision implicit in Rawls's unencumbered self – the ideal of a self-defining, self-realizing, and self-governing agent in the public sphere. In particular, full-time paid labour force participation for a "family wage" provided men, in principle, with the funds to support a dependent wife (and sometimes other domestic help) whose labour afforded them the time and flexibility to pursue self-selected economic and political objectives.

Given the centrality of breadwinning for male citizenship, the tendency for capitalist markets to leave some men bereft of the resources necessary for dignified labour force and civic participation evolved as the primary concern of the postwar liberal welfare regime. This concern informs the first pillar of the three-part framework for social citizenship that Rawls and Marshall proposed – the provision of social security. Over the first decades following 1945, family allowances, workers' compensation, employment insurance, pensions, and health care emerged as some of the most impressive policy achievements of the postwar welfare state. Each helped imperfectly to shield men's status as household breadwinners when job loss or diminished wage-earning capacities limited their abilities to provide financially for themselves and their dependants through market exchanges alone (for example, O'Connor 1993; Orloff 1993).

The theme of income security remained a dominant analytic lens for examining social citizenship well into the 1990s. For instance, in his influential book *The Three Worlds of Welfare Capitalism,* Esping-Andersen (1990, 3) claims that "the outstanding criterion for social rights must be the degree to which they permit people to make their living standards independent of pure market forces." This position motivated a contemporary comparative welfare regime literature in which it became common to describe the welfare state as an institution primarily interested in decommodifying citizens from the discipline of the market.

We saw in the previous chapter that neoliberals respond to the postwar emphasis on decommodification by arguing that policy went too far, resulting in hazardous dynamics that induce un(der)employed citizens to acquiesce to dependence on state provision. Feminists advance an alternative critique, although one that also acknowledges the importance of employment for social inclusion. In the feminist view, the postwar preoccupation with de-linking citizenry welfare from the dictates of the capitalist wage system distorts the fact that, before decommodification will be significant for individuals, they must first access the labour market. Historically, a primary welfare problem for many women has been too little commodification – not the converse presumed by Esping-Andersen's definition of social citizenship rights. His definition is, therefore, incomplete because it ignores that a key source of inequality in society rests with the fact that not all social groups are equally commodified (for example, Langan and Ostner 1991; O'Connor 1993).

The remedy, Orloff (1993, 318) argues, is to integrate into social citizenship analyses a "new analytic dimension that taps into the extent to which states promote or discourage women's paid employment – the right to be commodified."

At the heart of this feminist solution is the observation that securing a position in the paid labour force has emancipatory potential. This theme clearly resonates with neoliberal and third way proponents who urge the institutionalization of work responsibilities to encourage social integration among welfare benefit recipients. Although economic conservatives remain relatively disengaged with feminist research, Esping-Andersen's (1999, 2002) more recent work has gone a long way to integrate the insights of his feminist critics. The social investment state he now defends in the third way tradition explicitly rests on the concession that "the concept of decommodification is inoperable for many women unless welfare states, to begin with, help them become commodified" (1999, 44).

The feminist position that employment has emancipatory potential should give critics of welfare contractualism and the work (search) duties it implies reason to pause before simply discounting it as an example of miserly social policy. In fact, the Scandinavian welfare model, a beacon of light for many critics of neoliberalism residing in Anglo-liberal welfare regimes, is best seen as an "active entity, promoting reentry into the work force through retraining, and active involvement of women through the provision of publicly funded child care" (Cox 1998, 400). Underpinning Scandinavian activism, Cox explains, "is the idea that contributing to society is an obligation and duty of the individual. But because individuals often find it difficult to fulfill this obligation without assistance, Scandinavian welfare states help them" with supportive social programming (ibid.).

The relatively low level of poverty among lone-mother families in Sweden is one measure of the active welfare model's success. Compared to their counterparts in liberal welfare regimes, a much larger share of single mothers report market earnings as their main source of income. The result is that far fewer mother-only families encounter poverty-level incomes before social transfers in Sweden, compared to single mothers in the United States or Canada. The relative generosity of the Swedish welfare system, in turn, is far more effective than liberal welfare regimes at lifting out of poverty the much smaller share of lone mothers for whom employment does not preclude low-income status (for a more thorough discussion of this theme, see Sainsbury 1996, Chapter 4; Esping-Andersen 2002, 36-39).

The Principle of Reciprocity

The duty discourse in the Gilligan-motivated literature does not have paid work obligations as its primary focus when it argues that human interconnectedness implies mutual responsibilities. In fact, given Toronto's (1993, 166) concern that "the moral boundaries that surround a world constituted by the work ethic cannot recognize the importance of care," some may find counterintuitive the suggestion that the care ethic literature lends support for the institution of employment duties. Scholars working on the literature may go so far as to claim this suggestion actually subverts their intellectual objectives. However, in the light of the analytic thrust in feminism that ascribes to employment an emancipatory potential, the care ethic's concern with duties provides reason to contemplate at least the possibility that an ethically sound moral framework can integrate social obligations, including employment or active work search requirements, as a condition of receipt of social benefits.

Stuart White (2000) has been a leading scholar in developing this idea. He works within the tradition of T.H. Marshall (1964) to argue that the valuable insights about justice inherent in the social liberal paradigm are sufficiently malleable to integrate the idea of welfare contractualism. At a textual level, Marshall himself is open to this possibility. He affirms that, "if citizenship is invoked in the defence of rights, the corresponding duties of citizenship cannot be ignored. These do not require a man to sacrifice his individual liberty or to submit without question to every demand made by government. But they do require that his acts should be inspired by a lively sense of responsibility towards the welfare of the community" (112). Marshall goes on to discuss a number of citizenship obligations. Most notably, he argues that in order for the welfare state to be supported by a prosperous and growing economy, it must be supported morally and politically by citizens who put their hearts into their jobs and "work hard" (119). Marshall also cites a "duty to improve and civilize oneself ... because the social health of a society depends upon the civilization of its members" (82); "the duty to pay taxes and insurance contributions" (117); and the duty for organized labour to exercise industrial discipline so as not to disrupt with frequent strikes the success of the economy on which the welfare state depends (112).

White (2000) draws on this textual evidence to motivate his argument that the theoretical underpinnings of the social liberal paradigm do not unravel at the proposition that entitlement to social benefits should be made contingent on the discharge of social duties. Behind this concern, he notes, is the charge that welfare contractualism is incompatible with the idea of social rights that dominates Marshall's citizenship framework. Rights, the critique continues, "necessarily have a quality of unconditionality, and making the payment of welfare benefits which are notionally covered by a social right conditional on doing X or Y, as contractualism entails, apparently violates this necessary quality of unconditionality" (509).

The problem with this objection, White (2000, 510) observes, is that it fails to contemplate

> the distinction between: (1) a right to be given some resource, X, unconditionally; and, (2) an unconditional right of *reasonable access* to a given resource, X, where reasonable access means, in part, that the resource in question can be acquired and enjoyed by the individual concerned without unreasonable effort. A person can obviously have reasonable access to something, in this sense, without necessarily being directly given this thing. The notion of a social right can quite intelligibly be understood in the second way as well as in the first: as an unconditional right of reasonable access to a given resource, rather than as a right to be given this same resource unconditionally. This distinction is important ... because while welfare contractualism does seem incompatible with a social right of the first kind it is by no means necessarily incompatible with a social right of the second.

Rather than discredit the unconditionality of social entitlements, White (2000, 513) remarks that welfare contractualism has potential to represent an "expression of the ethic of solidarity" on which Marshall's and Rawls's liberal versions of egalitarianism rest. Explicit in the Budweiser™ model of social citizenship with which neoliberals sympathize is a principle of reciprocity: the idea that anyone who willingly shares in the mutual advantages made possible by society's cooperative venture has what White terms "a corresponding obligation to make a reasonable ... productive contribution to the community in return" (ibid.). The jingle "For all you do, this Bud's for you" captures this theme of reciprocity. It also implicitly acknowledges that we express our solidarity with fellow citizens who discharge their social obligations not only by offering assistance when they suffer significant hardship through no unreasonable fault of their own, but also by striving *not* to become a burden to fellow citizens when we personally can avoid this through reasonable means. "Free-riding on the provision of collectively enjoyed goods (including a collectively provided minimum income)," White concludes, is thus incompatible with the norms of reciprocity and mutual advantage that inform our intuitive understanding of social solidarity (ibid.). A society that strives to prevent free riding may, therefore, be working to enshrine the values of reciprocity and solidarity rather than undermining them.

While supportive of the reciprocity theme that is evident in neoliberalism, White goes on to improve Mead's version of the Budweiser™ model of citizenship by recognizing that the principle of reciprocity does not legitimately bind members of a community irrespective of the social conditions that characterize their society. This proviso is critical, since the neoliberal version risks subscribing to the "simply implausible" idea that "significantly disadvantaged individuals in a highly inegalitarian society may have an enforceable moral obligation to co-operate in their own exploitation" by being required to participate substantially in the absence of adequate recognition for their work (White 2000, 515). To defend against this risk, White argues that a principle of reciprocity can only be seen to legitimately oblige citizens when their community context satisfies four "intuitive conditions of fair reciprocity": (i) that a minimum standard of productive participation guarantees all citizens a decent share of the social product; (ii) that all citizens enjoy decent opportunities to engage in productive participation; (iii) that all citizens (capable of production) are enforced to comply with the minimum standard of productive participation; and (iv) that different forms of productive participation are treated equally (ibid.). (For a restatement of these conditions, see also White 2003, 134-37.)

The last of the four conditions raises the question: What should count as productive participation in society when evaluating whether someone is living up to the reciprocity principle? In his initial article on the subject, White (2000, 515) suggests that there is no reason to limit productive contributions exclusively to those performed in the formal economy when "society has two main institutions for social reproduction: the market and the family." In his subsequent book, *The Civic Minimum,* he gives only slightly more attention to this theme (White 2003, 108-13). White alludes to the often-repeated argument that "the raising of children has some features in common with public-goods provision," since the value of parenting work spills beyond the private family to the general public "because it helps to create the next generation of citizens" (110). Accordingly, he concludes that it is necessary to treat "some quantity of parental care as a form of civic labor ... allow[ing] it to ground claims to the social product, [and to] help ensure that the work involved in providing this particular public good is reciprocated

[so] that other citizens do not free-ride on the efforts of those who provide it" (110-11).

Ultimately, however, White sets the caregiving issue aside in favour of engaging more directly with neoliberals like Mead by discussing the extent to which their policy proposals are sensitive to the conditions in which it is fair to enforce labour market contributions. In this vein, he notes that many workfare programs in North America violate the first condition because they fail to ensure program participants reap a sufficient share of the social product (i.e., earnings) in return for their enforced social participation (White 2000, 515). Jurisdictions suffering high unemployment rates strain the second condition by severely limiting opportunities for productive labour market participation. The third condition supports policies that would tax inheritances and other wealth transfers to minimize the degree to which intergenerational exchanges allow some citizens to escape the expectation that they owe society a contribution through their own productive participation. As White (519-20) remarks, however, support for such tax measures is limited in Anglo-liberal countries, even outside economic conservative circles.

Although the modest attention that White gives his fourth condition for fair reciprocity will frustrate feminists working within the tradition of Gilligan, his defence of the principle of reciprocity nonetheless aligns closely with their interest in the mutual responsibilities implied by human interconnectedness. In fact, when his four intuitive conditions of fair reciprocity are examined through the lens of the care ethic literature, it becomes apparent that they raise considerations respecting the status of caregiving in society just as much as they stimulate discussions of employment. For instance, what would it look like for society to treat caregiving in the domestic sphere on a par with employment for the purposes of evaluating citizens' reciprocal contributions to society? What would it take to oblige all citizens, men as much as women, to share responsibility for caregiving equally when measuring the extent to which citizens reciprocate? And what societal restructuring is required to ensure that all citizens, men as much as women, have decent opportunities to contribute productively in their roles as caregivers for family and other close relations? These questions are at the heart of the Gilligan-inspired literature, and they motivate the discussions in the next chapters.

5
Premature Celebration

The celebration of the obliged citizen is premature despite the Idiot's acumen. No version of the duty discourse employed by neoliberals, the third way, communitarians, or social conservatives is adequate. They either overcompensate for social liberal permissiveness or embrace an incomplete understanding of social obligations that focuses on (ir)responsibility for employment without querying (ir)responsibility for caregiving. The problem in each case is that the duty discourses fail to engage adequately with feminist concerns about the patriarchal legacy of Western citizenship traditions.

Pateman (1989, Chapter 8) developed one of the first decisive analyses of this problem with her discussion of Wollstonecraft's dilemma. Her work illuminates the difficulties women still encounter in reaping the benefits associated with full membership in society because the citizenship ideal and practices that imbue our institutions originated with the premise that women would be excluded from many social spaces. Pateman's development of this theme, and the literature she motivated, guide the discussion in this chapter.

Scholars, including feminists, should be cautious when using citizenship as an analytic framework, Pateman warns, because dominant discourses present women with only two citizenry alternatives, neither of which facilitates dignified social inclusion. On one hand, she explains, women have demanded that the existing "ideal of citizenship be extended to them" in the pursuit of "a 'gender-neutral' social world" (1989, 197). On the other hand, "women have also insisted, often simultaneously, as did Mary Wollstonecraft, that *as women* they have specific capacities, talents, needs and concerns, so that the expression of their citizenship will be differentiated from that of men" (ibid.). Provision of unpaid care and welfare in the domestic sphere is presented by this second view "as women's work *as citizens,* just as their husbands' paid work is central to men's citizenship" (ibid.).

Both alternatives explored by Wollstonecraft are deficient because they acquiesce to patriarchal assumptions. The first implores women to "become (like) men" by pursuing full citizenship status through extensive participation in the labour market (Pateman 1989, 197). This option obfuscates important welfare contributions that women provide for no or little pay in private households and neglects the question of who will perform care work as more women assume increased earning responsibilities. By shielding the gender division of domestic labour from critical reassessment, the first citizenship route ignores that primary responsibility for care poses significant barriers to women's full participation in the labour market, civil society, and politics. Accordingly, Pateman concludes that, at best, the first option extends full citizenship status "to women only as lesser men" (ibid.).

In contrast, the second alternative acknowledges the intrinsic value of caregiving by rejecting the presumption that women should appropriate male citizenship patterns. Instead, it favours their retaining stronger attachment than men to the domestic sphere. This alternative offers few realistic strategies with which to defend against the economic disparity that the caregiver role suffers relative to the role performed by men in the paid workforce – a disparity that undermines the potential for the citizen-caregiver to achieve substantive equality with the citizen-breadwinner. Even were economic differences minimized, Pateman (1989, 197) notes that an exclusive caregiver citizenry option risks marginalizing women "as members of another sphere" separate from the market, civil society, and political arena.

Numerous scholars have grappled with the dilemma that Pateman identifies (for example, Cass 1994; Knijn and Kremer 1997; Lister 1997a, 1997b). Work by Fraser (1994, 1997) stands out for illuminating a path by which to break free from the intellectual shackles imposed by the dualism that constrains Wollstonecraft's choices. She argues against a vision of citizenship that subscribes to separate spheres for men and women, while also rejecting the androcentrism of the model that prescribes extensive labour market involvement for all citizens. The solution, she suggests, is a third option – what she refers to as the universal caregiver model of citizenship. Rather than expect women to approximate male standards or re-institutionalize their differential status, the third option would ask men and women alike to internalize the best of both models. In light of existing patterns of male privilege, the most pressing innovation requires the reorganization of social policy to induce far more men to modify their behaviour and attitudes to become more like most women today: people who shoulder considerable primary care work in addition to employment and other citizenry obligations and ambitions.

None of the duty discourses adopted by neoliberalism, the third way, communitarianism, or social conservatism manage successfully to transcend the dualism that defines Wollstonecraft's dilemma, although some communitarian and third way insights do suggest the need to move in this direction. Failure on this front makes their respective efforts to re-oblige citizens susceptible to various problems, including re-entrenching individualist predilections that undermine the potential for renewed interest in social obligations to champion the cause of reciprocity, as well as an impoverished vision of equality. I begin by exploring these issues as they arise in respect of neoliberalism.

Neoliberal Overcompensation

Neoliberals worry that the social liberal vision of the citizen as rights claimer risks undermining citizenry commitment to a principle of reciprocity. The focus on rights conveys a permissive attitude toward citizenship whereby individuals are entitled to make demands of others without necessarily making a productive contribution to society in return. The problem is so pervasive, neoliberals allege, that some citizens even fail to take reasonable measures to become financially self-sufficient through paid work in order to minimize their requests on the collectivity. The neoliberal remedy, we have seen, is to re-entrench employment obligations in social policy as a condition of welfare benefits, including for lone mothers, who represent a disproportionately large share of welfare recipients. This is the first citizenry alternative that Pateman contemplates, one that extends labour market expectations to all adults regardless of gender (although economic conservatives are not always consistent in applying this model to women outside low-income households).

The irony is that the neoliberal remedy for social liberal permissiveness overcompensates for the problem, with the result that it does just as much harm to the principle of reciprocity as does the liberal cousin it aims to improve upon. A preoccupation with promoting self-reliance through waged labour inclines neoliberal proponents to hold individuals personally responsible for their own economic difficulties. This approach to accounting for economic hardship reflects a propensity for individualist, decontextualized understandings of the sources of inequality, which risks submerging the "conditions of oppression, exploitation and inequality that determine when, how and which people can exercise 'individual responsibility'" (Kline 1997, 338).

This neoliberal shortcoming arises because its proponents prescribe a treatment for social liberal permissiveness without acknowledging that the problem stems from an indispensable theoretical insight. Marshall's and Rawls's emphasis on social rights reflects an appropriate sensitivity for the extent to which social, economic, and political opportunities are mediated by the distribution of primary social goods, as well as the tendency for market practices to exacerbate inequalities in the absence of state redistributive measures. An adequate solution to the permissiveness implied by the social liberal rights bias must, therefore, not ignore that, while people make choices, they do not always do so in circumstances of their own choosing. The range of alternatives from which we choose is embedded in and limited by the social, economic, political, and cultural environments that we inhabit, environments that advantage some far more than others.

Neoliberals, however, are reluctant to express sympathy for this social liberal insight given their commitment to free markets. Economic conservatives must downplay the influence exerted by social barriers when they explain poverty and other forms of discrimination so as to prevent debates over justice from interfering with the operations of the market. The result is that neoliberalism conceals from public scrutiny the role of the state and market in creating and reproducing relations of social and economic discrimination that contribute to poverty, ill health, joblessness, and exclusion for diverse groups of citizens.

Mead (1986, 69) exemplifies the tendency to individualize responsibility for inequality when he encourages skepticism about structural unemployment. In his view, "society's interest in work can be greater than the individual's, especially in the case of 'dirty,' low-paid jobs. For both rich and poor alike, work has become increasingly elective, and unemployment voluntary, because workers commonly have other sources of income, among them government programs. Jobseekers are seldom kept out of work for long by a literal lack of jobs. More often, they decline the available jobs as unsatisfactory, because of unrewarding pay and conditions." Mead maintains that a "pathological instability in holding jobs," rather than a dearth of employment opportunities, explains why many individuals are often without paid work (73). Employee turnover within low-skilled employment is difficult to blame on the economic environment, he suggests, since it is not influenced significantly by the ups and downs of the business cycle. Transfer dependency, he posits, is a more significant factor (76-82; see also Mead 1997b, 48-50; Murray 1987).

There is sound reason to resist Mead's doubt about involuntary joblessness, however. As Giddens (1994, 146-47) has observed, "if welfare incentives lead to underclass joblessness ... [this trend] should become reversed when welfare benefits decline, as they have done in many Western countries over the past twenty years. This has not happened." The Canadian case is an apt example. Over the past two decades, the Mulroney and Chrétien federal governments revised unemployment insurance by lengthening qualifying periods, reducing the duration and value of benefits, and disqualifying persons who "voluntarily" left jobs (for example, Evans 1997; McBride and Shields 1997, 91-96). Many provincial governments, in turn, reduced social assistance benefits significantly in the early and mid-1990s, led by Conservative governments in Alberta and Ontario, where cuts reached the 20 percent range (Kline 1997; Mayson 1999, 95). Despite these cuts, official national unemployment rates hover above 7 percent as of November 2004. Even if one grants that the decline from above 10 percent in the early 1990s indicates that citizens took several years to adjust to reorganized welfare incentives, the fact that unemployment persists around 7.5 percent despite six straight years of strong economic growth, lower benefit levels, and increased work and training obligations suggests that joblessness is due to much more than transfer dependency alone.

Despite the shortcomings of neoliberal analysis of unemployment, the recent cuts to social services and their reorientation around workfare imply a significant change in Canadian citizenship. Brodie (1995; 1996; 1997, 234-39), for instance, observes a new vision of neoliberal citizenship that embraces self-reliance, self-sufficiency, and the Protestant work ethic. Canadians are told that they must scale back their expectations of governments and accept a significant retreat in the scope and comprehensiveness of state-provided services. In place of universal state intervention, the citizenry is urged to assume the obligation to work longer and harder to take care of themselves and others so that governments can reorganize services to target only the "deserving" poor – persons who are unemployable due to disability or who demonstrate a sufficient commitment to the workforce but still earn subpoverty incomes.

This vision of citizenship rests on what Laycock (2002, 10) refers to as "a new story" by neoconservatives "about the people's enemies, a story based on a redefinition of 'special interests.'" Social movements on the political left formerly "portrayed as 'special interests,' opposed to the interests of 'the people,' various private-sector corporate groups and the political parties they funded" (ibid.). With the ascendance of neo-liberalism, however, economic conservatives have successfully redefined "special interests" in public discourse as "groups that support the welfare state, oppose major tax cuts, and propose that social resources should be allocated on the basis of non-market principles" (ibid.).

Richards's work on retooling the Canadian welfare state offers one example of the New Right tendency to pathologize so-called special interests. He argues that one of the "three disastrous syndromes" from which defenders of the postwar welfare regime suffer is "an unqualified identification with the claims of particular interest groups against society at large" (1997, 51). The expansion of the postwar welfare paradigm, he claims, was "accompanied by the growth of interest groups intent on defending specific programs. Their effect is to render extraordinarily difficult the exercise of Cabinet discretion – at either the federal or provincial level – in the field of social policy" (Richards 1994, 358). While Richards's indictment of interest groups focuses primarily on "public sector unions," "associations of contracted workers," "groups representing beneficiaries of major transfer programs," including seniors and seasonal workers, and "regional alliances in 'have-not' provinces" (359; Richards 1997, 175-84), he also singles out "women's groups" and organizations committed to promoting the rights of "gays and aboriginals" as contributing to the problem (1997, 54).

By disqualifying the legitimacy of special interests and their role in the policy-development process, Richards contributes to defending a citizenship ideal that depoliticizes social relations. In this view, the "good" citizen emerges as one who no longer seeks assistance from the state on grounds of systemic discrimination since it is assumed that one should be able to take care of oneself. As Workman (1996, 67) reports, activists who challenge government cutbacks on the grounds that they are harmful to welfare recipients, single mothers, and other disadvantaged groups are "dismissed as advocates of 'special interests,' a term calling attention to their refusal to accept the reasonableness of fiscal restraint on behalf of the entire social body." The resulting hostility toward special interests undermines the moral authority from which the disadvantaged can demand the redistribution of political and social power. As Laycock (2002, 43) warns: "Citizens who stop thinking that their personal challenges and problems are related to public decisions about justice make fewer demands for public support, and begin to believe that these private problems are essentially expressions of personal deficiencies, fate, or bad luck. When animated by a right-populist view of political life, such citizens are easily inclined to go even further and see the rights claims of others as self-interested claims made by 'special interests' against the people."

The conservative attack on special interests underpins what Laycock (2002, 10-11) describes as "a very effective campaign to redefine equality" in a way "that encourages 'ordinary' people to see themselves as victims of the machinations of special interests and state elites, neither of which can be effectively held accountable." So-called ordinary citizens are threatened by the inclusion of special interests in the policy arena because the former have "no such 'special' representation" (38). Special interests are thereby portrayed as asking to become "undeserving beneficiaries of ... state action" by deviating from an understanding of equality that would see "all citizens ... equally subject to the same laws, rules and benefits" regardless of the different circumstances that characterize their socioeconomic positions (10-11).

Jenson and Phillips (1996) have documented the effectiveness of this neoliberal critique of special interests on political practices in Canada. They report that both the Mulroney and Chrétien federal governments engaged in a "full-scale assault on the legitimacy and credibility of advocacy groups" under the guise "that the only legitimate representational form is a direct link between individuals and their MPs" (124). The consequences of this assault included the defunding of state institutions that nominally represented women's interests in the government, including the dismantling of the Canadian Advisory Council on the Status of Women. Spending cuts were also inflicted on the already minimally funded non-profit child care centres, women's shelters, and women's job training programs. The pejorative depiction of special interests further contributed to changes to the format of public consultations organized by federal and provincial governments, which now severely limit opportunities for group representation other than from a narrow set of business community voices (126-27; Laycock 2002, 36).

The retreat from (albeit inadequate) social liberal efforts to address the injustices inherent in divergent social and economic locations into which citizens are born in favour of a neoliberal preference for formal equality falls subject precisely to Pateman's critique of the first citizenship alternative contemplated by Wollstonecraft. The economic conservative hope that citizens can achieve equality and self-sufficiency through extensive commitments to waged labour discounts the important contributions that women have traditionally provided in private households at considerable cost to their own economic security, as well as the legitimate aspirations of many citizens to find sufficient time to participate fully in their domestic spaces. It also fails to think through sufficiently that women's disproportionate share of responsibility for caring for children and other dependants imposes considerable barriers to their working in paid employment for the hours that are necessary to sustain them and their dependants financially. I address these themes more systematically in the next section, in which I charge the duty discourses of neoliberalism, the third way, communitarianism, and social conservatism with being incomplete because they fail to adequately address caregiving obligations.

(Ir)responsibility for Care

The neoliberal focus on market discipline leads to analyses of social citizenship in which men's experience is the norm and the topic of caregiving is often marginalized. The result is that the neoliberal duty discourse fails to deal with the ubiquitous gender division of care and the problem of men's irresponsibility. In Canada, regardless of their employment status and occupation, women typically retain primary responsibility for work in the home, including caregiving. According to Statistics Canada (2000, 110), 94 percent of stay-at-home parents in single-earner couples are women. Women aged twenty-five to forty-four employed part-time are fifteen times more likely (32.5 percent versus 2.2 percent) than men of the same age to report that child care responsibilities preclude them from pursuing full-time positions (125). Women employed full-time typically remain responsible for organizing replacement care arrangements while they and their partners are in the labour force, as well as for coordinating the performance of domestic household work. Women employed full-time also consistently provide more unpaid caregiving than men employed full-time, and they enjoy less leisure on average than their male counterparts (Silver 2000).

The presence of preschool-age children particularly influences women's unpaid and paid workloads in a manner that diverges from the patterns of men. For instance, roughly half (51.1 percent) of full-time employed fathers in heterosexual relationships with a child under six provided fourteen or fewer hours of unpaid child care per week. In contrast, nearly half (48.7 percent) of mothers employed full-time with a child under six performed thirty or more hours of care weekly (Statistics Canada 1998). Almost all parental leave benefit recipients in Canada are women; just 11 percent were men in 2002 (Canada Employment Insurance Commission 2003, 18). Similarly, employed women with preschool children have twice the absenteeism rate due to personal/family-related responsibilities as employed men with children under six: women lost on average 3.4 workdays in 1999, whereas men lost only 1.8 days (Statistics Canada 1999a). This unequal division of care work means that women tend to perform far fewer hours of paid work, including in heterosexual households where both parents work full-time. Silver (2000, 27) reports that, in such households, mothers work roughly ten fewer paid hours a week than their partners. As the number of children in heterosexual two-parent households increases, the amount of paid work that mothers perform falls, while it increases for fathers (Drolet and Morissette 1997, 35).

Although women have adopted most of the roles formerly identified with the "male domain," the above data indicate that most men have yet to assume substantial responsibility for tasks historically identified as "women's work" in the domestic sphere. Research from the 1980s and 1990s suggests that most men in heterosexual relationships have not significantly increased the amount of unpaid household work they do, despite their partners' higher rates and longer hours of paid labour force participation (Beaujot 2000, 183; Conway 1997, 206; Phillips and Phillips 1993, 42). As Eichler (1997, 60) remarks, "there is a remarkable inelasticity in men's contributions to household tasks." Regardless of how much housework other women do on their behalf, men perform roughly the same amount. She notes that, "although there are some variations, the unequal division of [domestic] labour is not affected by social class, urban-rural differences, the number of children present in a household, whether or not the wife/mother is in the labour force ... or how many resources women have as measured in employment, education, reproductive decision making and family structure" (ibid.).

In light of this sort of data, the neoliberal interest in re-obliging citizens appears patently incomplete. It targets the relatively small pool of people who may be shirking employment expectations, while completely ignoring the much more prominent group of free riders that men of all classes represent when they neglect care and other domestic labour. Taylor-Goodby (1991, 201-2) puts the point this way:

Care-work, reproductive labour, is vital to the continuance of society. Even those who are prepared to disallow the claims of the frail elderly and others who are incapable of contributing to future productivity must see the upbringing of the new generation as indispensable to social existence through time ... The whole sexual division of labour appears to function as a vast engine of moral hazard, in which perverse incentives encourage one sex to refuse to participate in a major division of the totality of social labour. If welfare rights discourage a small number of people of limited employability from seeking paid employment, that is one thing. If the operation of the welfare state discourages the male half of the population from playing an equal role in the fundamental task of social care it is a much more serious problem.

Neoliberals are not alone in showing insufficient concern for the issue of moral hazard as it is implicated in the gender division of care. The problem also plagues social conservatives, third way proponents, and communitarians to some extent.

Communitarians Diagnose but Cannot Fix the Problem

Of the non-feminist discourses so far considered, communitarians like Etzioni (1993, Chapter 2) come closest to acknowledging the problem of male irresponsibility for care. This acknowledgment is implicit in his allegation that there is a parenting deficit that sees children suffer from a dearth of parental involvement from both mothers and fathers. His position that "few people who advocated equal rights for women favoured a society in which sexual equality would mean a society in which all adults would act like men, who in the past were relatively inattentive to children" (63) closely echoes Fraser's (1994) analysis. Similar to her universal caregiver proposal, Etzioni (1993, 63) recommends that we should transcend the dualism that defines Wollstonecraft's dilemma by advocating a "new gender-equalized world" that combines "all that was sound and ennobling in the traditional roles of women and men," one in which "men would be free to show emotion, care and domestic commitment," just as women would be free to work any place they wish.

The strength of Etzioni's diagnosis of the problem is not matched by an equally sophisticated analysis of how to actually oblige men to care more in domestic contexts and share responsibility for caregiving more equally with women. His cursory references to parental leave benefits, telework, and part-time employment leave unexplored the economic and cultural factors that induce heterosexual couples to approximate the primary caregiver/primary breadwinner division of labour, particularly following the birth of a child. While I explore these issues in more detail in Chapter 7, it is worth noting that the gender earnings gap remains significant in Canada, despite high female labour force participation rates in international terms. Statistics Canada (2000, 141) reports that women who work full-time, full-year, earn on average 73 percent of male earnings. So long as the large majority of heterosexual women continue to earn less than male partners, Becker's (1981) classic joint-decision model of household behaviour reveals that it is rational for the spousal unit that wants to maximize household income to decide that the woman will reduce paid work or drop out of the labour market completely to rear children. This household dynamic is the origin of a cycle of dependency that drives many women into economic insecurity and dependence on a male partner, while pushing fathers to commit to longer employment hours and dependence on female caring (Slaughter 1995).

Even within households where the earnings gap is minimal or actually favours the female partner, pervasive cultural norms about gender exert considerable influence over the decisions that individuals make regarding care and employment. As Olson (2002, 392) aptly remarks, since personal "dispositions are patterned along lines of gender, men and women will to some extent reproduce the normative cultural background of their socialization. The choices they make [about caring and earning], in other words, will express not only what is rational in a self-interested sense, but equally important, what it means to be a man or woman in their society." Unfortunately, Etzioni's discussion of paternal responsibilities skirts the complexity implicit in the economic and cultural factors that reproduce the gender division of labour. The result is that his Pollyannaish policy proposals fail to acknowledge that women represent seven in ten part-time workers and that women almost always take leave benefits in liberal welfare regimes. Etzioni's suggestions, therefore, get us no closer to obliging men to care.

Conservatives Are Mired in Wollstonecraft's Dilemma
Although Etzioni offers no adequate remedy to male irresponsibility for care work, at least he alludes to the problem. The same cannot be said for economic and social conservatives. Instead, these political camps typically ignore the problem by retreating to the two models of citizenship that define Wollstonecraft's dilemma. We saw in Chapter 3 that Mead and Richards affirm a gender division of care labour when they discuss households that are not dependent on income assistance, a theme that is consistent with Wollstonecraft's second option. Social conservatives express a similar sentiment. For instance, in Canada, Smith (1997) recommends tax-policy changes to permit women who work in the home to be paid a salary by their husbands. She also advocates that homemakers be added to the official list of professions so that mothers would become eligible for unemployment insurance as "working women," as well as eligible to make contributions to the Canada or Quebec Pension Plans (ibid.). Smith's proposal is one that subscribes to what Fraser (1994,

605-6) refers to as the "caregiver parity model," which has as its aim "not to make women's lives the same as men's," but rather to mitigate the costs associated with women's different role. In this view, "child-bearing, childrearing, and informal domestic labor are to be elevated to parity with formal paid labor. The caregiver role is to be put on a par with the breadwinner role – so that women and men can enjoy equivalent levels of dignity and well-being" (606).

The assumption of role complementarity that undergirds the caregiver parity model is also explicit when social conservatives raise the concept of paternal duties. Gilder (1987), we have seen, argues that fatherlessness is a particularly deleterious social trend, the solution for which is to reassert male breadwinning responsibilities and to re-domesticate women, including low-income mothers. Popenoe (1996), a more sophisticated social conservative, aims to accommodate some female employment when discussing fathers' responsibilities, but his analysis nevertheless develops from within a distinctly patriarchal framework. For instance, his extensive anthropological and biological discussions convey an overzealous sympathy for gender essentialism. The result is that he often portrays the involved father as a mother's helper in regard to child care and the person who retains patriarchal power as family head and the voice of reason. In fact, Popenoe's ideal father strongly resembles the model evoked in preachings by the evangelical Christian Promise Keepers movement in the United States, which urges men to acknowledge that they are equal to, but different from, their wives. In this vision of equality, husbands are encouraged to assume the spiritual leadership role in their families, which they fulfill by serving their wife and children, in part through the performance of household tasks and child care (Silverstein et al. 1999).

Gender role complementarity, even when promoted with rhetorical flourishes urging new financial supports for women at home, is subject to a litany of problems that render it an unacceptable foundation for both gender equality and household income security. To begin with, efforts to compensate women for their care labour run aground on questions of implementation and valuation (Maloney 1989, 194-95). If the value of domestic care is determined by reference to what it would cost to replace in the market, any strategy to compensate unpaid caregiving would appropriate a market-based system of valuation that operates in a context in which women already provide a significant amount of care for no pay. Research on gender wage differentials suggests that some female-dominated jobs pay less, in part because they resemble, if not compete with, the kind of work that women do for no wage at home

(Gaskell 1991; Teghtsoonian 1997, 124). Any appeal to the market to determine the rate of compensation for currently unpaid labour would, therefore, invoke a system of valuation premised on the power dynamics that the proposed compensation is meant to counter.

In addition, proposals to provide a homemaker's wage are financially untenable. If it is assumed that spouses will pay for the domestic work from which they benefit, the proposal completely disregards the circumstances of unemployed and low-income spouses who do not have the income to pay wages. It also neglects the situation of lone parents who shoulder substantial careloads in addition to employment responsibilities. Who will pay for their care work? If the state is expected to substitute for spouses, Phillips and Phillips (1993, 150) estimate that such a proposal could cost Canadian governments at least $30 billion annually.

Since a wage system is a non-starter fiscally, proponents of the view that a gender-differentiated citizenship model could be refurbished to minimize the costs of unpaid domestic labour are resigned to accept less expensive measures. Smith's recommendation of pension reform is one option that receives attention in feminist literature (Phillips and Phillips 1993, 156-59). Pension reform may be a helpful short-term measure to mitigate the costs for women who specialized in domesticity in keeping with earlier social expectations. In particular, enriched pensions for mothers could alleviate some of the poverty that continues to plague senior unattached women in Canada at rates higher than their male counterparts (Statistics Canada 2000, 137). Ultimately, however, pensions that are not indexed to earnings are highly unlikely to garner the long-term public support necessary to ensure their payments approximate earnings-based schemes. The result is that pensions for mothers will rank caregiving as a second-tier citizen occupation by delivering benefits that are considerably less valuable than those attainable in the labour force.

The tax system is another tool often referred to as a potential mechanism to financially compensate women's unpaid care labour. However, tax proposals typically amount to little more than symbolic recognition. For instance, the Canadian Income Tax Act, section 118(1)(c.1), currently permits a $560 caregiver tax credit for persons who support an elderly dependent relative. Similarly, the Reform/Alliance Party advocated in 1999 for the conversion of the Child Care Expense Deduction into a refundable tax credit that would deliver approximately an additional $1,200 per child to stay-at-home parents (Coyne 1999; McCarthy 1999a, 1999b). Although the total bill for this proposal would have been several billion dollars, the effects would be modest for individual mothers, since an extra thousand dollars or so is insufficient to mitigate the economic dependence that accompanies specialization in domesticity.

The problems with the caregiver parity model are not simply implementation issues, however. Policy models based on complementarity and specialized activities for women and men are subject to an implausible essentialism that depicts all women as naturally inclined and contented nurturers, ignoring the various ways in which women and men differ in this respect (Lister 1997b, 18). In addition, while one can imagine that wages or pensions for mothers might render women "independent, well provided for, well rested, and respected" in their specialized citizenry domain (Fraser 1994, 599), Fraser echoes Pateman's concern about social marginalization by pointing out that women would nonetheless remain "enclaved in a separate domestic sphere, removed from the life of the larger society" (ibid.). Although caregiving work is a critical source of welfare and satisfaction for individuals, families, and communities, this work is not appropriately valued if its performance necessitates the marginalization of caregivers from other important social spaces and sources of fulfillment, such as "in employment, in politics ... [and] in the associational life of civil society" (ibid.). Full community membership implies participation across important areas of social life, including, but not exclusively, the domestic sphere.

A gender-differentiated model of citizenship also demeans caregiving work since it does not value it sufficiently "to demand that men do it too" (Fraser 1994, 609-10). The model includes no expectation that men amend their behaviour and practices to recognize and contribute to the welfare potential associated with care work. Nor does the model acknowledge unpaid care ambitions among men. One result is that it risks further marginalizing men away from the domestic domain, where the opportunity to nurture children, spouses, relatives, and other intimate relations holds out rich emotional and psychological rewards that can shape one's sense of self, history, belonging, and purpose. This risk is particularly worrisome in light of new research about fathers, which shows that men regularly identify (at least rhetorically) their becoming a father as the most important event in their lives and exhibit a desire to diverge from the parenting practices of absent fathers (Coltrane 1996, 118-21).

The inadequacies of the parity model continue in respect of income security, both among individual women and households. The model obfuscates the significant financial insecurity to which exclusive caregivers are subject since this role entails that they forgo employment income and employment benefits, suffer a depreciation of their human capital and employment marketability, and relinquish opportunities for training, wage raises, career advancement, and enriched pensions. Although the risks inherent in forfeiting their economic independence may appear acceptable (and "rational" from the standpoint of the couple) so long as at-home caregivers reside with their spouse, the risks frequently materialize for women in the form of significantly lower living standards or poverty when a couple divorces or a partner dies (Armstrong 1997, 42-43; Eichler 1997, 36). In 1999, 41.3 percent of single-mother families with children under eighteen had after-tax household incomes that fell below Statistics Canada's low-income cut-offs (LICOs), a rate many times higher than that of couples (National Council of Welfare 2002, section 7). Although some single mothers who leave married or common-law relationships escape poverty, almost all experience a significant drop in their standard of living, while their ex-spouse regularly enjoys a noticeable improvement. In addition, the traditionally high rates of poverty among unattached women over sixty-five reflect the economic legacy of extensive commitments to unpaid caregiving, as well as lesser pension entitlements that accompany this domestic role. Despite policy changes that have significantly reduced the poverty rate among women seniors from 38 percent in 1980 to 22 percent in 1998 (National Council of Welfare 2000, Figure 7.14), many older women continue to live below or near the poverty line, and the share of women over sixty-five who suffer low-income status in Canada is twice the share of men in the same demographic category (Statistics Canada 2000, 137).

When we turn attention to household security, we are reminded that female employment increased enormously over the past three decades not only in response to a cultural transition regarding the appropriate role for women, but also to compensate for declining real wages for men. Findings from Beaudry and Green (2000) indicate that successive waves of labour market entrants since the 1970s, particularly men, have consistently fared poorly in comparison to earlier entrants, regardless of education levels. The real decline in starting wages is significant: a university-educated male entrant in 1992 earned approximately 20 percent less than his counterpart did twenty years earlier, and he is not eventually compensated for his lower initial wages by increasing returns for experience. The result is that Canadian households today must perform considerably more paid labour per year (typically by a second adult) in order to enjoy a level of economic well-being and security earned by the one-earner family that was much more prevalent thirty years ago. The implication is that the parity model's nostalgia for the one-earner family is anachronistic. Statistics Canada (2000, 146) data confirm that the percentage of dual-earner families with low income in 1997 would have been much higher in the absence of earnings contributed by wives, rising from 4.7 percent to 17.5 percent.

While retaining a relatively strict gender division of care labour represents an inadequate foundation for citizenship, the other alternative that conservatives support – extensive labour market attachment for all citizens premised on male employment norms – is also problematic. Fraser (1994, 604) refers to this alternative, illuminated by Wollstonecraft's dilemma, as the universal breadwinner model. "It aims to achieve gender equity principally by promoting women's employment. The point is to enable women to support themselves and their families through their own wage earning. The breadwinner role is to be universalized, in sum, so that women too can be citizen-workers," as has been the cultural expectation of most men of working age since the Second World War.

An affinity for the universal breadwinner model guides Courchene's (1994a) proposals to restructure the Canadian welfare state. His concern about transfer dependency resonates with the feminist interest in reorganizing policy analysis so that it integrates a new analytic dimension that monitors the degree to which state institutional arrangements encourage or discourage employment. The emphasis he places on education, training, and workfare also implies that social security should no longer be viewed primarily as protection from market operations but, instead, as a system that nurtures one's capacity to participate in, and adapt to, markets that shift in response to global pressures.

Given this vision of security, Courchene acknowledges the importance of child care as a key social program for the postindustrial social and economic order insofar as it prepares citizens for, and facilitates their participation in, the labour market. In his view, "day care is a policy whose time has finally arrived. It is much easier to rationalize day care in the emerging knowledge-based society than in the former resource-based society, since one can argue for human capital formation on the part of parents and children alike. However, it is a big ticket item and the only way that we can probably afford even a limited system is in the context of a wholesale restructuring of the existing social envelope" (Courchene 1994a, 82).

Courchene offers little detail of the child care system he envisions, especially in terms of the labour force needs of women. His most recent discussion of child care proposes "A Human Capital 'Bill of Rights' for Children" (2001, 163). The bill would insist that "access to childcare/

daycare should become the right of every child by virtue of Canadian citizenship and not restricted by either income class or whether both spouses are gainfully employed" (167). He recommends a "daycare voucher" system that would entitle children to participate in developmental programs premised on age-appropriate educational curriculum along the lines of "Dr. Maria Montessori's impressive model" (164). But Courchene is ultimately silent about a number of issues that are critical to overcoming employment barriers for mothers, including the age at which children would become eligible to claim the universal benefit, the number of days per week that children would be entitled to care, the time of day that care would be available, or any associated fees. This lack of attention to elements of a child care system that are integral to women's employment reflects Courchene's (1994a, 80) view that "a move to universal day care, as in the Scandinavian countries will not trigger a major increase in labour force participation of females: they are already in the labour force."

Implicit in Courchene's position is the assumption that most Canadian women have managed to arrange adequate strategies for shouldering employment and caregiving in the absence of significant public assistance. The problem with this assumption is that it runs ahead of reality. While Canada has relatively high female labour force participation rates in international terms, the full-time dual-earner family with children is only the "seeming norm," to borrow a phrase from Beaujot (2000, 230). Data from Canada's National Longitudinal Survey of Children and Youth (Ross, Scott, and Kelly 1996) indicate that the majority of children under twelve in two-parent families reside in homes that remain neotraditional. The survey found that 36 percent of such children live with parents who both work full-time, compared to 33 percent who have at least one parent who is not employed, and 22 percent who have at least one parent employed part-time (ibid., Table 3.10). Given that stay-at-home parents are overwhelmingly mothers, and that women constitute 70 percent of part-time workers, these data suggest that a large share of heterosexual two-adult homes are dividing paid and unpaid work along patriarchal lines when children are under twelve. This division of labour sustains the primary earner/secondary earner dynamic, generating costs that are just as significant for women today as they were several decades ago.

Costs include the sizable gender earnings gap that has already been discussed. The gender earnings ratio reveals that the average woman in Canada earns 64 percent of what the average male does when part-time and full-time workers are considered. This finding reflects that women disproportionately labour in shorter-hour employment contexts, often due to their need to accommodate more caregiving responsibilities than men (Statistics Canada 2000, 141, 111, 103). Actual work experience is another significant explanatory factor in Canada. According to Drolet (2002a), interruptions in women's labour force participation for child-rearing purposes contribute more significantly to the earnings gap than do differences between women and men in educational attainment, areas of specialization, and supervisory responsibilities.

Another significant shortcoming of Courchene's analysis is that it overlooks the stress, and related health implications associated with role overload, that is a principal affliction suffered by full-time employees today, particularly women. Canada's 1998 General Social Survey (Statistics Canada 1999c) found that 38 percent of married women aged twenty-five to forty-four who were employed full-time report high levels of stress, as did one-quarter of married men. The rate of high stress rises to 50 percent for women employed full-time with a child under five, as well as among lone mothers (ibid.). Studies suggest that stress levels are particularly high for mothers because they continue to bear primary responsibility for unpaid childrearing tasks (Brisson et al. 1999). Although the demands of the modern workplace often raise blood pressure rates for both men and women, research shows that these rates regularly drop to normal levels for most men after work. In contrast, a study by University of Laval researchers indicates that blood pressure levels for many women remain elevated well after the paid workday, a reality that significantly increases their risk of stroke and heart disease (ibid.). In particular, the Laval study found a strong correlation between women's high blood pressure during off-work hours and a lack of support from male partners with childrearing responsibilities.

The source of Courchene's misguided analysis of child care is a standard economic conservative assumption, one captured by Eichler (1997) in her discussion of the "individual responsibility model of the family" (see also Lewis 2001). Eichler observes that the policy trend which increasingly portrays women as citizen-(wage) workers reflects the assumption that women are capable of fulfilling *either* the care *or* the provider functions. But within a neoliberal policy context preoccupied with self-reliance, this assumption yields a perverse effect. From the assumption that one person is capable of *either* role, "the conclusion is drawn that *one* parent should be able to do both" (Eichler 1997, 13-14). This leap in logic assumes away the extensive labour inherent in domestic and caregiving obligations, which pose barriers for many women to overcome before they can commit to the labour market to the same degree as many men, and which compound their stress levels when they opt for full-time employment. It also sets the ideological stage for the containment, and in many cases erosion, of public supports for citizens' caregiving ambitions and obligations, despite the rapid decline in time available for households to perform domestic responsibilities. The assumption of individual responsibility allows neoliberals to reconcile, at least intellectually, the tension inherent in their desire to prioritize citizenry labour force participation while simultaneously restraining state expenditures on new child care programs, as well as cutting expenditures in other social care policy domains. Neoliberal cost cutting and program redesign have been documented by an extensive Canadian literature (for example, Bakker 1996; Evans and Wekerle 1997; McBride and Shields 1997). This research reveals that governments substantially reduced public expenditure on health care, child welfare, child care, and other services in the 1980s and 1990s on the assumption that families (read women) would pick up the slack irrespective of higher female employment rates.

The risk implicit in Courchene's assumption of individual responsibility was made manifest most recently in policy decisions in British Columbia. The Government of British Columbia (2002, 4) has redesigned eligibility for social assistance among single parents. Legislation now requires "employable" lone parents to seek work when their youngest child turns three, down from age seven. The aim of the new policy is to reduce social assistance caseloads by requiring lone parents to capitalize more on the welfare potential of labour markets, in keeping with a broader reorientation of social services around the concept of workfare. However, the government has simultaneously restricted eligibility for provincial child care subsidies by lowering the income level under which low-income citizens qualify for public child care assistance (Kershaw 2004). Given the province's position that employment is the best social program, the decision to cut child care subsidies for low-income parents is difficult to comprehend in the absence of the individual responsibility model, since it exacerbates the challenges that child care costs pose for single parents trying to find and retain employment.

The Third Way: A New (but Still Inadequate) Gender Contract

Third way proponents also advocate a universal breadwinner vision. They depart from economic conservatives, however, by rejecting the individual responsibility model of the family in favour of what Esping-Andersen (2002, Chapter 3) terms a "new gender contract" (see also Giddens 1999, 94-95). In Esping-Andersen's (2002, 69) view, gender equality must now be recognized as "a 'societal affair,' a precondition for making the clock-work of postindustrial societies tick." With this concession he signals the substantial influence that feminist critiques have had on his theorizing since he first published his influential welfare regime typology in *The Three Worlds of Welfare Capitalism* (1990). Integrating insights by Orloff (1993) and others, he accepts that a welfare state suitable for the postindustrial era must feature a universal system of child care premised on Scandinavian levels of public investment that reduce parental fees to no more than roughly one-third the actual cost of quality care so that barriers to female employment are significantly reduced (Esping-Andersen 2002, Chapter 2).

Esping-Andersen's (2002) case for gender equality and child care is couched primarily in efficiency terms as a foundation for his strategy to combat welfare risks that concentrate in young households. "Women's paid employment emerges as a key ingredient in any strategy to combat poverty in child families" (30), he maintains, since the costs of their interrupting work for family reasons are compounded over the life cycle due to "skills erosion, less experience, and lost seniority" (86). These penalties on women's earnings potential influence not only their own life-course chances, but also their children's, since "it is well established that the ability and motivation to learn in the first place depends on the economic and social conditions of childhood" (9). He therefore identifies greater access to quality child care, which facilitates maternal employment and ensures sufficient intellectual stimulation for children when their parents are at paid work, as a "proactive investment against family and market welfare failure" that can prevent the deleterious consequences for child development that correlate with household poverty (Esping-Andersen 1999, 164). "There is one basic finding that overshadows all others," he indicates: "That remedial policies for adults are a poor (and costly) substitute for interventions in childhood" (2002, 49). He thus concludes that affirming and facilitating the symbiotic relationship between child welfare and female employment is "*sine qua non* for a sustainable, efficient, and competitive knowledge-based production system" (28).

As part of its new gender contract, the third way engages to some extent with the issue of male irresponsibility for care. Giddens (1999, 89-98), for instance, speaks of democratizing the family, which implies a "shared responsibility for child care, especially greater sharing among women and men, and among parents and non-parents, since in the society at large mothers are bearing a disproportionate share of the costs (and enjoying a disproportionate share of the emotional rewards) of children" (94-95). Similarly, Esping-Andersen (2002, 70) observes that "the egalitarian challenge is unlikely to find resolution unless, simultaneously, the male life course becomes more 'feminine.' In other words, if we want more gender equality our policies may have to concentrate on men's behaviour."

Like Etzioni, however, Giddens does not supplement his discussion of the democratic family with careful policy analysis. While he urges family-friendly workplace policies, his proposals are cursory at best, making brief mention of telework, work sabbaticals, and paid family leave to supplement child care (1999, 125-26; 2000, 48). No mention is made of the fact that, at present in liberal welfare regimes, fathers rarely take advantage of such benefits to reduce their paid work schedules for the purpose of caring for children or other dependants.

In contrast, Esping-Andersen (2002) develops a more sophisticated analysis of parental leave systems, in which he concedes the low take-up rates among men cross-nationally. He therefore finds that there is good reason to "question whether parental leave incentives for fathers actually make much of a difference" to the amount of care work that men perform (93). If obliging fathers to care is a societal priority, he concludes that a much more "substantial alteration of the male incentive structure" is necessary since "it appears unlikely that even the most progressive parental leave policy, alone, will make a huge difference" (ibid.).

Esping-Andersen does not follow up this recognition, however, by investigating further what is required to alter the incentive structure in which men make choices between care and employment. Instead, he minimizes the extent to which male life patterns require feminization. The crux of his most recent research retains strong sympathy for the social liberal analytic approach that portrays care and connection as impediments to autonomy and independence, without acknowledging that they are sometimes also sources of protection and fulfillment. The result is that Esping-Andersen regards the domestic sphere predominantly as something for citizens to overcome. "Clearly," he states, "mothers' employment prospects (and the family economy) would be better served by daycare than by encouraging fathers to put in more unpaid hours. Policies that advocate more male participation within the household may appear egalitarian from a gender point of view, but they do not appear to be a 'win-win' strategy. Most households, we can assume, *would prefer to reduce the necessary unpaid hours for both partners if that were possible*" (Esping-Andersen 1999, 59-60; italics added).

The presumption that citizens are better off when they overcome domesticity reveals important limits to the reach of feminist analysis in

Esping-Andersen's latest research. His sympathy for the idea that social inclusion is found in employment indicates a willingness to accommodate primarily those aspects of feminist analysis that pose the least challenge to the male model of citizenship, while remaining resistant to elements of feminist research that require a more dramatic departure from androcentric assumptions. This does not deny that his recognition of the unequal commodification of some groups of women represents a substantial improvement over his analysis in *The Three Worlds of Welfare Capitalism*. Rather, the point is that this facet of feminist analysis is only one (albeit a very important) aspect of its critique of mainstream welfare research. Esping-Andersen's vision neglects the second integral element, which is concerned with properly valuing the informal care that is performed in the domestic sphere. Care is portrayed by many feminists as both labour and love, a site of exploitation and, just as importantly, satisfaction, in keeping with the essential ambivalence of human connection that is observed in the care ethic literature. Exploitation must be acknowledged in light of the unequal sexual division of care that poses a barrier to women's autonomy. But this exploitation does not ultimately negate what Elshtain (1981, 333) refers to as the "humanizing imperative" of the activity, its importance for social reproduction, labour supply, and economic growth, nor the fulfillment that citizens may derive through care provision.

The new third way gender contract thus remains inadequate. While its commitment to universal child care makes a valuable contribution to debates about welfare recalibration, it nonetheless retains too strong a connection to the universal breadwinner model. Theorists who remain committed to this model by presenting domesticity as something for citizens to escape on the path to inclusion fail to appreciate that time for care in one's domestic spaces is an essential element of social belonging. The vital role of private time for social inclusion is the subject of Chapter 6.

6
Private Time for Social Inclusion

As a normative objective, social inclusion presupposes an answer to the question "Inclusion where?" The dominant answer in policy and social science circles assumes that participation in the paid labour force is sufficient for achieving inclusion. This vision informs Esping-Andersen's (2002) latest version of the social investment state. As he puts it, "paid employment remains, as always, the basic foundation of household welfare and it is hardly surprising that more jobs are seen as the *sine qua non* in the pursuit of an inclusive society" (21).

The purpose of this chapter is to challenge the dominant assumption that citizens must escape domesticity to achieve social inclusion. I will argue that obstacles to participation in one's network of intimate familial and fictive kin relations are just as much impediments to the practices of full social membership as are barriers to inclusion in the labour market. This position amounts to another version of "The personal is political," with which feminists critique the public/private divide. I am arguing that the domestic sphere, which is often treated as the most private of citizenry spaces, must be recognized as an important sociopolitical domain for the purposes of promoting inclusion.

The support I marshal for this position relies importantly on insights offered by feminist theorists who place the experiences of women of colour, especially African American women, at the centre of their research. The feminist scholar Collins (1991, 1994) has been particularly successful at demonstrating that motherhood is intimately implicated in identity politics and issues of individual and collective power. But, as she points out, "these themes remain muted when the mothering experiences of women of color are marginalized in feminist theorizing" (1994, 61). In response, she and Roberts (1995b) urge feminists to reconstruct the dominant view of motherhood by integrating the circumstances of ethnic minority women into their research, rather than simply appending them. The analysis in this chapter contributes to this reconstruction.

By linking the issues of social inclusion and domestic caregiving, I also aim to mine the motherhood re-theorization project initiated by Collins and Roberts for resources it can contribute to the broader feminist concern to develop a concept of citizenship that rejects the citizen-worker model in favour of a model in which the social citizen is both carer and worker (for example, Fraser 1994; Lister 1997a). The focus on race and ethnicity, in addition to gender and class, that I bring to this broader objective is consistent with work by Williams (1995), who was among the first scholars to supplement gender critiques of Esping-Andersen's typology with a critique that more thoroughly illuminates his omission of issues concerning both race and gender. As part of this research, Williams outlines a framework for comparative welfare regime analysis that incorporates the themes of inclusion and exclusion as they pertain to the disparate spheres of family, work, and nation (149). While issues of inclusion are not the primary focus of her article, Williams's framework nonetheless suggests the value of a project that examines more carefully the relationships between participation in kin networks and inclusion in other social contexts.

Integrating the Experiences of Women of Colour into Citizenship Theory

The assumption that women must transcend domesticity to achieve gender equality fails to engage with the racial and classist social dynamics that mediate the experience of domestic caregiving for diverse groups of women. Analytic perspectives that are sensitive to these dynamics reveal that the social ideal of devotion to domesticity that was ideologically ascribed to white, class-privileged women has been, and remains, circumscribed by barriers that limit the access of some poor, ethnic minority, and immigrant women to their own domestic spaces. These barriers position many such women to regard more time for domestic care as a critical element of their emancipation, rather than as their principal site of social exclusion (Dua 1999, 242; Misra and Akins 1998, 274-75). As a first step in challenging the dominant view about social inclusion, I therefore return to this line of feminist literature to explain why some marginalized women express a desire for more domestic time. This literature identifies three related sets of barriers that frustrate some women: state legislation, ideology, and financial need.

One example of state legislation that limits access to domestic spaces is found in the history of immigration in Canada which, as in other countries, is replete with policy decisions that institutionalized considerable barriers to family life for select groups of women and men. British colonial settlement strategies and later Canadian immigration practices were informed by the overarching goal of creating a white settler nation (Arat-Koc 1997, 74; A.B. Bakan and Stasiulis 1997b, 33). When they were tolerated before the 1960s, men and women of colour were permitted to migrate to Canada predominantly in response to capitalist demands for low-cost labourers. The demand for cheap labour first increased considerably in the late nineteenth century as the Canadian economy advanced toward industrialization. Difficulties attracting British and European immigrants compelled the state to supply Canadian employers with labour via migration from China, India, and Japan. Dua (1999, 244) observes that, "in the context of a white, settler policy and the politics of racial purity, Asian migrants were defined as temporary workers rather than potential citizens of Canada." Governments imposed a differential residency and citizenship status on Asians, denying them the right to vote, naturalization, ownership of certain kinds of property, access to some occupations, and, until 1947, equal opportunity to sponsor spouses and children. As a result, the majority of Asian migrants were men, many of whom were forced to leave behind their wives and offspring. This enforced separation meant that "the demand for a 'family' became a central issue" in minority ethnic communities as members struggled to resist the Canadian state's denial of their right to live in a family context of their choosing (245).

The struggle of some women of colour for more time to care in familial domains is also a response to ideological forces that devalue their motherwork. The (dis)organization of families of colour by early immigration policy reflects how the ideal of female devotion to domesticity includes not only an image of the "good" mother, but also images of women who are allegedly less suited for motherhood due to their social location amidst relations of race, class, and other identity-related characteristics, including marital status (Kline 1995, 121). The series of externally imposed controlling images of African American womanhood identified by Collins (1991, 70-78) provides a useful analytic tool by which to illuminate ideological processes that disqualify some marginalized women from the status of "good" mothers. This disqualification, in turn, engenders within some women the desire to resist social stereotyping by performing care work in their own domestic spaces (Roberts 1995b, 204).

The dominant ideal of exclusive motherhood ideologically distanced single and working-class women of all ethnic backgrounds from the path to citizenship integration available to women in more financially advantaged households. Economic need meant many single and low-income women were confronted by a context of choice that precluded the option of remaining home full-time (Boris 1994, 176). Unable to rely solely on a man's earning power, such women were required to balance the double day of paid work and informal domestic labour long before the term became popularized in contemporary thinking. Exacerbating their heavy workload, they also risked social condemnation as women who allegedly neglected their domestic responsibilities because of their labour force participation.

Collins (1991, 74-75) captures this social dynamic in her discussion of the Black mother matriarch image. This cultural image "contends that African American women fail to fulfill their traditional 'womanly' duties. Spending too much time away from home, these working mothers ostensibly cannot properly supervise their children and are a major contributing factor to their children's school failure" (74). The labour attachment highlighted by the matriarch metaphor portrays Black motherhood as deviant because it "challenges the patriarchal assumptions underpinning the construct of the ideal 'family'" (75). Consistent with views proffered by social conservatives like Gilder (1987), Collins (1991, 74) argues that Black mothers are portrayed as "overly aggressive, unfeminine women ... [who] allegedly emasculate their lovers and husbands. These men, understandably, either desert their partners or refuse to marry the mothers of their children." The effect of the matriarch image is to blame social ills that afflict families of colour on "bad" mothers who deviate from feminine norms established by privileged white policy makers.

Although ideologically disqualified from the category of "good" mothers, many poor and working-class women have historically been recruited for low-paid work as caregivers in white, economically privileged homes (Glenn 1994; Roberts 1995a, 230). Between 1871 and 1941, domestic employees constituted the single largest category of paid female workers in Canada (Fudge 1997, 121). Work in private households has been an especially important source of employment for women of colour (Arat-Koc 1997, 73).

Long hours in domestic work historically limited the capacity of many women in this occupation to care personally for their families (Roberts 1995a, 235), thereby positioning this group to serve as forecasters for the modern experience of work-family conflict that has become the norm for many women in Canada and the United States. The frustration that such women report about their estrangement from their own domestic spaces is often especially acute because domestic workers are expected to sacrifice nurturing their own kin in order to care generously for, and integrate within, their employer's family (Dua 1999, 247). Collins (1991, 71) examines this tension in her discussion of the cultural image of the Black mammy, who was expected by white male power to love, nurture, and care for "her white children and 'family' better than her own." Collins explains that, "no matter how loved they were by their white 'families,' Black women domestic workers remained poor because they were economically exploited. The restructured post-World War II economy in which African American women moved from service in private homes to jobs in the low-paid service sector has produced comparable economic exploitation. Removing Black women's labor from African American families and exploiting it denies Black extended family units the benefits of either decent wages or Black women's unpaid labor in their homes" (72).

The family sacrifices that Collins aligns with long hours at the periphery of the labour market are exacerbated by immigration legislation that institutionalizes an extreme degree of estrangement from intimate relations for foreign domestics – Canada's modern mammies. Under the Live-In Caregiver Program (LCP), foreign domestics, predominantly Filipino women, enter Canada on temporary employment visas. They are eligible to apply for landed immigrant status only after performing two years of domestic work for a designated employer. During this period the foreign domestic must live with, and work exclusively for, her employer-family, and she has no standing to sponsor her own children or spouse to immigrate to Canada (A.B. Bakan and Stasiulis 1997a, 20).

The LCP received front-page news attention in 1999 and 2000 in Canada when foreign domestic worker Leticia Cables received a deportation order. The problem, as reported by the *Globe and Mail,* was that "she work[ed] at too many jobs" (Leblanc 1999). Ms. Cables contravened immigration law for foreign domestics by accepting extra caregiving and housecleaning work with families in addition to the family named on her employment authorization. "Immigration officials ... said her breach of the rules might take away work from Canadians and was serious enough to scotch her chances of getting landed-immigrant status for her and her husband and two teenaged children, who still live in the Philippines" (Mitchell and Laghi 2000). Ms. Cables's circumstances thus reflect the ongoing commodification of some immigrant women of colour as workers – before mothers – by Canadian immigration policy. Foreign domestics are recruited to perform work that Canadians are unwilling to do. But when recruits endeavour to compete for jobs that Canadians may seek, the LCP implies that they are no longer welcome in Canada, nor are their families.

When paid work proves unavailable or insufficient to shield their families from economic deprivation, poor mothers can approach the welfare state as clients of social assistance, eligible in liberal and conservative welfare regimes for the least generous and most stigmatized social benefits (O'Connor 1993, 504; Orloff 1993, 315; Sainsbury 1996, 129-47). In many cases poor mothers are subject to social and legal scrutiny, including regulation by child welfare law through which the dominant ideology of motherhood wields considerable power to discipline women. Kline (1995) reports that the acts or omissions of poor women that diverge from the dominant motherhood ideal are routinely decontextualized from the realities of racism, colonialism, immigration, violence, and classism during child welfare and other regulatory proceedings in which women are evaluated in terms of their suitability as mothers. The resulting disproportionate separation of mother and child among minority ethnic families, particularly among Aboriginal families in the Canadian context, can be perceived as an example of societal devaluation of kin relations within communities of colour.

Roberts (1995b) develops a parallel argument about the disruption of kin relations within African American families by linking the recent policy shift to promote workfare for lone parents with the cultural metaphor of the Black welfare mother – a third externally imposed controlling image of African American womanhood identified by Collins (1991, 76-77). Whereas the matriarch image constructs Black women as "bad" mothers because they are overly aggressive in the male sphere of paid work, the welfare mother metaphor identifies Black women as "bad" mothers because they are not aggressive enough. Instead, with the aid of social assistance, the Black welfare mother "is portrayed as being content to sit around and collect welfare, shunning work and passing on her bad values to her offspring" (77).

Roberts (1995b, 200) explains that many contemporary US welfare reformers have "in mind" the image of the Black welfare mother when they devise remedies to respond to heightened concern about growing welfare dependence. In the past, when public assistance benefited predominantly white women, the ideology of exclusive motherhood historically supported the delivery of financial aid to lone mothers on the grounds that they should not relinquish their domestic duties as caregivers. Roberts notes that "the mothers' pensions of the Progressive Era benefited almost exclusively white mothers: only 3 per cent of recipients were African American" (200-1). In the contemporary context, however, she argues that maternalist rhetoric no longer has sufficient political influence to sustain public social assistance for stay-at-home single mothers, in part because "the public views this support as benefiting primarily black mothers" (200). Maternalist rhetoric holds less sway, she contends, because "many workfare advocates fail to see the benefit in poor black mothers' care for their young children." Instead, consistent with welfare critiques advanced by Mead (1986), "payments to these mothers [are thought to] encourage transgenerational pathology that perpetuates poverty" (Roberts 1995b, 201; see also Mink 2002).

The social depreciation of some women's caregiving, their ideological disqualification from the status of "good" mothers, and the far-reaching legacy of racism in immigration policy remind social scientists that we should not take for granted the capacity to have and support a family of one's choosing. The interaction of discriminatory public policy and the unequal distribution of socioeconomic resources (both intra- and internationally) produce obstacles to domestic participation that disproportionately impede some social groups more than others.

Concern about socioeconomic factors that undermine citizens' abilities to form and support families has received some attention beyond research circles that organize theorizing explicitly around issues of race. The work of Orloff (1993) offers one instructive example. Her initial effort to rework Esping-Andersen's approach to social citizenship not only supplemented his focus on decommodification with an analytic dimension concerned with access to paid work; it also articulated a dimension attuned to "the capacity to form and maintain autonomous households." Orloff's treatment of this second dimension originally emphasized the need to guarantee "those who do most of the domestic and caring work – almost all women – ... [the ability] to survive and support their children without having to marry to gain access to breadwinners' income" (319). Her concern in this first formulation is to free women from the bonds of marriage or cohabitation with men when such relations are abusive or no longer desired. But the capacity to maintain autonomous households entails more than women's independence. It also directly addresses the question of whether women or men enjoy the necessary social circumstances to establish families that will thrive. Orloff speaks to this other question in her more recent collaboration with Monson (2002). They argue that the capacity to form an autonomous household "gets at whether women and men are allowed to have as well as to support families, thus reflecting the character of regulations of sexuality, custody, reproduction, marriage, divorce and household composition. We might call this *access to family*, or the 'right to a family'" (68).

Interest in the "right to a family" is evident even in recent work by Esping-Andersen in the context of his discussion of fertility. While his principal interest is the labour supply needed to support an aging population (Esping-Andersen 1999, 67-68), he also worries about the disjuncture between the number of children that citizens indicate they desire and actual fertility rates, which are typically lower. In his view, "the ability of citizens, in the first place, to form families according to their true aspirations must be regarded as the bottom-line measure of any society's welfare performance" (Esping-Andersen 2002, 63). The concern in this instance "is not the long historical decline in fertility, nor pronatalistic objectives, but simply families' apparent inability to arrive at desired welfare levels. Hence, we must be concerned with the obstacles that citizens face in forming families of their choosing" (ibid.).

The claim that "the bottom-line measure of any society's welfare performance" is a citizen's capacity to form families according to her or his aspirations is a powerful insight for theorists of social inclusion to contemplate. Although Esping-Andersen does not integrate this insight into his theorizing to the extent that it dampens his sympathy for the dominant vision of inclusion as participation in the paid labour force, his failure on this front should not be seen as an example for other researchers to follow.

Participation in One's Domestic Sphere Is a Necessary Condition for Social Inclusion

The previous section examined reasons to resist constructing domesticity only as a site from which women must escape on the path toward equality and inclusion. The discussion of barriers to family life locates the issue of domestic participation as part of the broader issue of the politics of time. A wide range of public policy decisions concerning immigration, social assistance, taxation, labour standards, parental leave, and child care mediates the access that citizens enjoy to both paid and unpaid temporal opportunities. Lister (1997a, 201) has observed that "*time* is a resource for citizenship ... which is generally highly skewed in favour of men." The discussion so far in this chapter supplements her observation by showing that, in addition to gender, there are race and class underpinnings to the politics of time as it influences individuals' opportunities to enjoy family life.

But does the recognition that time for care in the domestic sphere is a political matter mean it is also an issue that pertains to social inclusion? The latter arguably refers only to participation in important community spaces – not private households or family and other intimate networks. Some may worry that appending questions of family time to the social inclusion debate risks extending the reach of the inclusion concept so far that it loses its utility as an analytic dimension.

With due concern to preserve the utility of the inclusion concept, I believe this sort of skepticism about extending its purview to include questions of domesticity should be resisted. In this section I aim to defend the position that time to care in one's domestic sphere is a constitutive element of community membership, at least within communities defined by a shared ethnicity or faith background. Put somewhat differently, I argue that the realm of the sociopolitical must include the domestic for the purposes of promoting social inclusion in pluralist societies. The support for this position draws on the theme of resistance that pervades theorizing about the motherwork of women of colour.

Domesticity as a Site of Refuge, Resistance, and Belonging

T.H. Marshall's (1964, 72) classic definition of "the whole range" of rights associated with citizenship's social element includes "the right to share to the full in the social heritage." However, in pluralist societies the social heritage of members of minority ethnic and faith-based communities is often absent in public spaces. Members of gay and lesbian communities also risk a similar kind of social isolation in public spaces that fail to affirm their sexuality. Rather than enjoying recognition of their heritage and identity in the public sphere, members of these marginalized social groups often experience persecution, violence, labour exploitation, misrecognition, and systemic discrimination. Against this public backdrop, one's network of familial and fictive kin relations emerges as a sphere in which individuals can find a reprieve from some forces of oppression. The search for this reprieve underscores why theorists who focus on the circumstances of communities of colour often portray the sphere of family as "a refuge against racism" (Dua 1999, 242), "a site of solace and resistance against white oppression" (Roberts 1995a, 236).

The themes of survival and protection that pervade Collins's (1991, 1994) research about motherhood reveal that the refuge offered by domestic spaces can be a deadly serious matter for members of ethnic minority communities who confront social realities where their own survival, as well as that of their children, has historically been (and in some cases continues to be) threatened. She explains that the care performed by some poor and minority ethnic women represents "mothers fighting for the physical survival both of their own biological children and those of the larger ... community" (Collins 1994, 50), as well as the right to retain custody of wanted children amidst a child welfare system that imposes culturally biased standards (53-54; see also Kline 1995; Mink 2002, 122-23; Roberts 1995a, 231). In this context, African American mothers are said to "place a strong emphasis on protection, either by trying to shield their daughters as long as possible from the penalties attached to their race, class and gender status or by teaching them skills of independence and self-reliance so that they will be able to protect themselves" (Collins 1991, 126). Fostering familial survival thus becomes "a form of resistance" for some minority ethnic mothers (140) whose reproductive and care labour on behalf of their own families defies the expectation of servitude to whites (Roberts 1995a, 236).

In addition to survival and protection, a construction of domesticity as a site of solace illuminates how individuals often discover and cultivate within this sphere the kinds of intimate relationships that are constitutive of social belonging. Family and fictive kin not only provide material assistance when times are difficult, but they can also provide important emotional support by affirming personal values and self-definitions. As Gray (2000, 25-26) remarks, "in order to flourish most people need social support for their values and identities." Since this recognition may be lacking in public domains for members of minority ethnic and faith-based groups, as well as gay and lesbian communities, the positive recognition of one's self-definition that can be found in domestic spaces grows in significance. In this instance, domesticity assumes the status of an essential sphere of social belonging, where the nurturing of one's identity assists individuals to resist externally imposed denigrating images, including the cultural metaphors of mammy, matriarch, and welfare mother discussed above. The web of relations in which citizens provide and receive care in domestic spaces thus becomes what Collins (1991, 118) describes as a site where members of marginalized social groups "express and learn the power of self-definition, the importance of valuing and respecting ourselves, the necessity of self-reliance and independence, and a belief in [our] empowerment."

Recognition that time for familial relations can protect individuals from material deprivation and social isolation is consistent with the origin of the term "exclusion" in French political debates, which, as Esping-Andersen (2002, 29-30) indicates, is the intellectual source of the term "social exclusion." Martin (1996, 382) observes that French thinkers initially aligned the risk of exclusion with "two phenomena which combine and reinforce each other." The first, from which the received view about inclusion now draws heavily, is the risk of being left out of the labour market or employment. But the second parallels closely the line of analysis in this chapter: namely, the "risk of seeing one's network of social relations and primary integration broken up because basic social links, of which the family link is the most important, disintegrate." Thus, in contrast to the now dominant approach to inclusion, the original French debate gave considerable attention to "relational vulnerability" (ibid.), which acknowledged that exclusion can result from loss of contact with "network[s] of integration" that extend well beyond employment contacts (386). Martin (382-83) notes that concern for relational vulnerability is consistent with the theme of social capital that emerged out of the work of Bourdieu (1980) and now receives extensive attention in literature associated with Putnam (2000). This analytic tradition recognizes that citizens' involvement "in a network of family, neighbourhood, association, [and/or] friendships" can act "as a catalyst for their social 'capital' ... This network is simultaneously a source of information, protection, support and mutual help" (Martin 1996, 385). The loss of primary integration in domestic settings is, therefore, significant because "it involves losing a sense of protection, mutual aid and support through such means as exchange, gifts, barter, and other features of the informal economy" (388).

Domesticity and Identity Politics

The links between family participation and social capital that are evident in the French tradition lend strong support for reintegrating into the dominant view of social inclusion the recognition that domesticity is an important domain when questions of social inclusion are at issue. But the French tradition as described by Martin (1996) ignores an equally significant reason for rethinking the inclusion debate in this manner – namely, the role of domestic caregiving in the politics of identity and recognition. This issue again is implicit in Collins's treatment of the relationship between resistance and motherhood.

The identification of domesticity as a potential refuge acknowledged that motherwork can be a site of self-definition in which some minority ethnic women resist externally imposed denigrating images. In this section I examine what Collins (1994, 49) refers to as "the significance of self-definition in constructing individual and collective racial identity." A proud sense of self that is indexed to a strong attachment to one's ethnic heritage positions some women of colour to function as cultural workers within their families and broader communities. The care that some women in minority ethnic groups provide in their domestic spaces contributes significantly to the development of a sense of self-worth among the children in their care. The failure of schools, the media, and other public institutions to validate the identities of racialized ethnic groups requires that mothers compensate by shouldering what Roberts (1995a, 225) describes as "the incredible task of guarding their children's identity against innumerable messages that brand them as less than human." The care work of minority ethnic mothers thus encompasses the responsibility to cultivate "a meaningful racial identity in children within a society that denigrates people of color" (Collins 1994, 57). Mothers must teach their children "to survive in systems that oppress them," while ensuring that this survival does "not come at the expense of self-esteem" (ibid.). By instilling within children the confidence to trust their own self-definitions and values, minority ethnic mothers equip their offspring with "a powerful tool for resisting oppression" (Collins 1991, 51).

The emphasis that Collins places on fostering self-esteem converges with the primacy that Rawls assigns to this theme in his seminal work. For Rawls (1971, 440), "the most important primary good" is self-respect, which he defines as having two parts. The first "includes a person's sense of his own value, his secure conviction that his conception of his good, his plan of life, is worth carrying out" (ibid.). The second includes "confidence in one's ability, so far as it is within one's power, to fulfill one's intentions" (ibid.). Without these two qualities, Rawls observes, "nothing may seem worth doing, or if some things have value for us, we lack the will to strive for them. All desire and activity becomes empty and vain and we sink into apathy and cynicism" (ibid.). Wary of the kinds of constraints on agency that Rawls attributes to self-doubt, Collins's treatment of motherhood reveals that care performed by some minority ethnic women assumes as one purpose the prevention of apathy and cynicism among children whose self-worth is not necessarily validated in public structures.

The struggle of some minority ethnic women to instill within their children a proud ethnocultural awareness reveals that their "subjective experience of ... motherhood is inextricably linked to the sociocultural concern of racial ethnic communities – one does not exist without the other," Collins (1994, 47) observes. This insight suggests that domestic care has the potential to function as a form of resistance to oppression that stretches well beyond the particular homes in which the work is performed because it contributes to a broader project of community development. *Qua* cultural workers, mothers contribute significantly to the project of "group survival" by transmitting an ethnocentric worldview to the next generation (ibid.; Collins 1991, 145-54). Collins (1991, 143) attributes the survival of certain African customs in North

America to the conscious effort made by Black women to preserve specific traditions. This observation draws attention to the role served by women from minority ethnic groups as cultural conduits in polyethnic countries such as Canada and the United States, which have been built on immigration. By working to ensure that children cultivate a proud affiliation with their cultural history, ethnic minority mothers help to preserve the distinctness of the minority collective racial identity.

Kymlicka (1989) indicates the importance of securing this collective identity in his defence of minority rights from within the liberal tradition of Rawls. Despite the careful attention that Rawls gives to the relationship between self-respect and agency, Kymlicka observes that he fails to demonstrate sufficient concern for the source(s) from which people derive the beliefs about value around which they develop meaning and self-respect in their lives. This inattention is problematic, Kymlicka explains, because our selection of values and life pursuits by which we express our agency "is always a matter of selecting what we believe to be most valuable from the various options available, selecting from a context of choice which provides us with different ways of life" (164). The context of choice within which we operate is "determined by our cultural heritage. Different ways of life are not simply different patterns of physical movements. The physical movements only have meaning to us because they are identified as having significance by our *culture*, because they fit into some pattern of activities which is culturally recognized as a way of leading one's life" (165).

Consistent with Collins's focus on motherhood, Kymlicka (1989, 165) adds that we learn about these patterns of activity starting with the care we receive in our earliest years: "From childhood on, we become aware both that we are already participants in certain forms of life (familial, religious, sexual, educational, etc.), and that there are other ways of life which offer alternative models and roles that we may, in time, come to endorse. We decide how to lead our lives by situating ourselves in these cultural narratives, by adopting roles that have struck us as worthwhile ones, as ones worth living (which may, of course, include the roles we were brought up to occupy)."

The goal of cultural survival with which Collins aligns motherhood finds some support in one strand of social inclusion literature that argues: "The adequacy and coherence of contemporary agenda of social inclusion require their engagement with the politics of difference" (Stewart 2000, 5; see also Lister 2000b, 44). Indicative of this literature, Ratcliffe (2000, 177) encourages an interpretation of inclusivity that "involves an acceptance of the right of any individual/community to maintain a 'minority identity' which is different/distinct (from that of the 'majority society') in religious and cultural terms whilst at the same time retaining full citizenship rights, in a Marshallian sense." Research on motherhood that builds on the work of Collins intersects with this literature about inclusion and difference by making explicit the connection between minority identity and a critical context in which identity is shaped. Collins (1991, 1994) goes to great lengths to demonstrate that analytic perspectives sensitive to race and ethnicity expose how care provided and received within one's web of familial and other intimate relations is integral to the development of self- and community definition. In this manner, her analysis re-invokes the dialogical thesis of human agency, identity formation, and self-understanding around which communitarians, social conservatives, and feminists working in the tradition of Gilligan converge, as we saw in Chapter 3.

The dialogical character of agency has significant policy implications for states intent on institutionalizing commitments to social inclusion that will facilitate the maintenance of minority identities. Public policy must recognize that the time citizens have for care in their domestic spaces can be essential for the transmission, preservation, and definition of ethnocultural identity. This time for kin caregiving may be especially important for social groups that cannot count on their collective identity being institutionalized and positively represented in public spaces. To borrow language from Kymlicka (1989, 190), public validation of the dominant identity provides "for free" to members of this privileged ethnocultural group what marginalized minorities have to "pay for: secure cultural membership." The theme of this chapter is that minority groups do not just pay for this security; they also *care* for it.

The relationship between caring and group membership remains muted in theorizing that reflects dominant ethnocultural perspectives where the collective identity is not at risk. But relative silence does not mean that time for domestic care is any less critical for the development of identity among members of the dominant culture. The dialogical character of agency is as much a reality of identity formation in privileged sociocultural groups as it is in marginalized communities. Domestic care is an activity that facilitates individuals, regardless of their privilege, to explore their place in a family and community lineage as well as the values and life pursuits that this social location affirms. Thus, although the dialogical thesis illuminates the importance of domestic care as a form of resistance among some minority sociocultural groups, it also underscores the broader point that informal caregiving is integral to identity formation among all citizens, irrespective of the security of their ethnocultural background. Private time for care is, therefore, an issue of identity politics that commands attention from us all.

Domesticity, Power, and the Sphere of the Sociopolitical

Recognition of the domestic sphere as a locus of identity politics and belonging where refuge may (potentially) be found from oppression or economic misfortune turns the public/private divide inside out. Contra dominant liberal and civic republican traditions, this recognition propels domesticity into the realm of the sociopolitical for the purposes of evaluating and facilitating social inclusion. Processes of identity formation that unfold in domestic spaces are crucial for understanding the ability of some individuals and the social groups in which they are members to claim and exercise power in welfare states. This insight provides further evidence for the view that "'any definition of "political participation" is inevitably tendentious and contestable,' given that the drawing of the line between the political and the non-political is itself a political act" (Parry, Moyser, and Day 1992, 20). Collins (1991, 140-41) lends support for this conclusion when she critiques traditional social science approaches to civic activism. She notes that "white male conceptualizations of the political process produce definitions of power, activism, and resistance that fail to capture the meaning of these concepts in Black women's lives ... For example, conflict approaches to social class see labor unions and political parties – two modes of political activism dominated by white males – as the two fundamental mechanisms for working class activism. African American women have been excluded from both of these arenas, leaving conflict models bereft of a theoretical analysis of Black women's social class protest."

This whitewashing of some activism research fails to acknowledge that "unofficial, private, and seemingly invisible spheres of life and organization" provide spaces that can be just as important for some social groups' political resistance as are the formal domains of political contest that are the subject of most academic inquiry (Collins 1991, 140). Depending on their access to traditional culture, Collins observes that domestic and other family spaces are available for African American women "to create Black female spheres of influence, authority, and power that produc[e] a worldview markedly different from that advanced by the dominant group" (147). Within this sphere of influence, the political projects of resistance and cultural survival are initiated.

The sociopolitical character of domesticity may be more prominent in African American circles because this sphere is not aligned exclusively with the nuclear family. Since long hours in labour markets denied many women of colour the role of exclusive mother, alternative institutional arrangements evolved in Black communities "to resolve the tensions between maternal separation due to employment and the needs of dependent children" (Collins 1994, 51; see also Roberts 1995a, 235). Women in extended family structures, fictive kin, and neighbours often assumed additional responsibilities as "othermothers" for children regardless of blood relations (Collins 1991, 119-23). One result is that domesticity for such women regularly encompassed public elements in light of their caring for members of the community in addition to persons with whom they shared a home.

In part because their care work transforms the public/private divide, caregiving by some ethnic minority women emerges as a public symbol and source of empowerment. Collins (1994, 55-56) reports that "many Black women receive respect and recognition within their local communities for innovative and practical approaches not only to mothering their own 'blood' children, but also to being othermothers to the children in their extended family networks, and those in the community overall." By "fostering ... community development" and "furthering the community's well-being," care work in some minority ethnic communities establishes a "basis for community-based power," which in turn establishes othermothers as "powerful figures" within local networks (56). Roberts (1995b, 204) adds that "concern for children has often served as the foundation for formal collective struggles among African American women, such as the Sisterhood of Black Single Mothers in Brooklyn and the Welfare Mothers' Movement. It may be that the experience of communal mothering has led some black women to become community activists in order to make a better life for the entire community's children. Black women often explain their involvement in social activism as an outgrowth of their experience as mothers."

The argument that the boundaries of the sociopolitical should be broadened to include some caregiving performed in domestic spaces pushes the limits of what even some of the most stalwart feminist supporters of redefining political participation have so far been willing to concede. For instance, Lister (1997a, 29) advocates a vision of the "public sphere" that "pertains not just to the arenas of formal politics," but also to "the myriad of voluntary associations of civil society, most particularly the kinds of campaigning and community groups in which women are most likely to be active." In keeping with Putnam's work about social capital, Lister (2000a, 42) observes that the "grassroots networks and organizations" that evolve out of political action at the neighbourhood level are "a prerequisite for effective public policy" and "an expression of healthy citizenship." Like Collins, Lister regards small-scale political participation as an important source of empowerment and "self-confidence" for individual women, which "is a prerequisite for effective citizenship" (ibid.).

Nonetheless, Lister (2000a, 43) ultimately resists embracing domestic spaces as sites of active social and political citizenship. She maintains that "the argument that motherhood (and, from a contemporary stance, other forms of care) should be treated as the equivalent of more public duties as a criterion of citizenship made more sense in the context of the struggle for the basic political right of female suffrage than it does now in relation to the conceptualization of active political citizenship" (49).

The arguments of this chapter, however, challenge Lister to rethink this position and broaden her vision of the sociopolitical further. Once the sphere of the family and other fictive kin relations is recognized as a significant domain for identity politics, as well as for refuge, resistance, and activism, a definition of active citizenship that excludes domesticity entirely from the terrain of citizenship becomes less tenable.

This proposed re-envisioning of the realm of the sociopolitical is not without risks. The depiction of domesticity as a potential site of social inclusion does not mean that it is also a site where social cohesion is nurtured. Any treatment of domesticity as a sociopolitical space in which time to participate is defended on the ground that it is a primary location for identity politics, where ethnocentric worldviews can be preserved and transmitted, risks supporting socialization processes that foster social divisions. As Kymlicka and Norman (2000, 35) warn, "it is surely true that if ethnic, regional, or religious identities crowd out a common citizenship identity, there will be difficulty maintaining a healthy democracy."

Social Inclusion Entails a Right to Time for Care in Domestic Spaces
Notwithstanding this concern about social cohesion, the recognition that domesticity is a locus for social belonging and identity politics lends strong support for institutionalizing what Knijn and Kremer (1997, 332) have described as "the right to time for care" so that citizens enjoy adequate opportunities to participate in the group membership practices that occur in family and fictive kin settings. Knijn and Kremer treat this right as a constitutive element of "inclusive citizenship" (ibid.). This citizenship vision, they argue, "should be based on the assumption that every citizen, whether male or female, could claim the right to give care to people in his or her immediate context when circumstances demand it. The notion of citizenship should contain the idea that every

citizen at some time or another has to take care of people they care about. At some point within a citizen's life, people have to care for young children, and at other times close friends or elderly parents need personal care" (331).

There is an interesting parallel between this approach to inclusion and Esping-Andersen's (2002, Chapter 2) shift in favour of viewing "a child-centred social investment strategy" as an indispensable foundation for his new vision of welfare states. Part of his defence of this vision rests with his depiction of "families" as "the key to social inclusion and a competitive knowledge economy" (29). Motivated by a central concern to ensure that citizens are not "trapped in inferior life chances," Esping-Andersen argues that "it is essential that we focus our lens on childhood and family welfare" since "all evidence indicates that (early) childhood is the critical point at which people's life courses are shaped" (30).

It is important to recognize how Esping-Andersen's interest in families, as it pertains to issues of social inclusion, differs from an understanding of inclusion premised on a right to time for care in domestic spaces. The latter engages directly with individuals' interests and pursuits, recognizing that many citizens will aspire in some circumstances to care for others in a family setting for one or more reasons, including the search for a site of solace, resistance, and identity preservation, which has been discussed in detail in this chapter. Such a desire may reflect aspects of a person's self-understanding as a parent, a loved one, and/or a member of a certain community.

In contrast, Esping-Andersen (2002, 9) identifies the family as an arena for inclusion primarily because the care that people perform there has the potential to prevent exclusion among, and foster the human capital of, members of the next generation. Thus, when Esping-Andersen is not treating care in domestic settings primarily as an impediment to women's autonomy, he regards it principally as a public resource for promoting efficiency that the state should capitalize on – not as an individual project or pursuit that also holds out the possibility for citizens to find satisfaction and belonging, as well as a site of political struggle in some cases. The result is that Esping-Andersen only superficially investigates how to facilitate domestic time for parents to provide "cognitive stimulation" by indicating that "one option ... is to ensure that [they] are given the possibility of low-stress employment and adequate time with their children" (49). But since he ultimately recognizes that "we cannot pass laws that force parents to read to their children," he suggests that "we can compensate" by promoting the "more effective option" of "universal, high quality day care" (ibid.), an option which sidesteps the issue that citizens often desire to care personally.

It is well acknowledged in feminist literature that women's caregiving is a resource that governments, labour markets, and men exploit. However, many feminists are careful not to treat care simply as an instrumental resource; they resist the assimilation of care into what Elshtain (1981, 333) refers to as the realm of "shitwork," which, wherever possible, should be minimized. In the social inclusion literature this resistance is evident in work by Levitas (1998), who alludes to the value of integrating citizenry care aspirations into the social inclusion debate. She notes that extant political discourses pay little attention "to the ways in which paid work may impede inclusion" (169). One example she offers is that long hours in the labour force render parents unable "to collect young children from school" (ibid.). This lack of time "affects participation in the social networks that develop around the school and in the neighbourhood as well as the relationship between parent and child" (ibid.). She thus concludes that "paid work leaves less time for many other activities" that contribute to social inclusion, including some unpaid work (ibid.).

Levitas's treatment of informal care as an important issue for social inclusion is weakened, however, by her tendency to equate unpaid work with caregiving. The analysis in this chapter warns against treating the two as equivalent, at least in the context of social inclusion debates. It is not dusting or ironing work that renders domesticity an important locus for belonging and the transmission of ethnocultural identity; it is diverse forms of care by which family, fictive kin, and sometimes community members nurture one another physically, intellectually, emotionally, politically, and/or spiritually. Nor, as Jenson (1997b, 183) points out, should it be assumed that care work within the family is always unpaid: "This work may well be paid, as it is in regimes with close-to-replacement rates for caring leaves, as in the Nordic countries. Or it may be minimally reimbursed, as it is when leaves are low-paid, flat rates (as French parental leaves are) or when 'recognition' of child raising is compensated in pension regimes at the lowest rates (again, as in France)." Consistent with Jenson's insight, I argue in Chapter 7 that the issue of payment becomes a critical factor when institutionalizing a right to time for care in the domestic sphere that will challenge, rather than entrench, the patriarchal division of labour.

Aligning the pursuit of social inclusion with a right to time for care (rather than with unpaid work) in domestic spaces also engages directly with the research of Fraser (1994) on women's citizenship. We have seen that she responds to Wollstonecraft's dilemma by arguing for the need to overcome the androcentric character of citizenship that underpins the worker-citizen model in the dominant discourse about inclusion. Public recognition that time for domestic care is a necessary element for the achievement of social inclusion would substantially weaken the grip of masculinist norms on citizenship practices. Consistent with Fraser's vision, this recognition would move society a long way toward treating "human beings who can give birth and who often care for relatives and friends" not as "exceptions," but as "ideal-typical participants" in society (599-600).

Time for Care, Women's Autonomy, and Public Policy Challenges

The finding that social inclusion comprises time for domestic care raises a number of challenging public policy questions. Two questions are: How much time to care informally in one's domestic domain is required for the purpose of achieving inclusion? And how can we embrace domestic time as a critical element of social inclusion without reinforcing the patriarchal division of labour?

The first question concedes that time for care in one's network of intimate relations is a necessary, but not sufficient, condition for inclusion. The arguments of this chapter are meant to supplement, not replace, the more exhaustive attention that has been devoted to the issue of women's right to be commodified. Time for informal care must not crowd out time for labour force participation, which is typically the most significant source of financial welfare and economic security in citizens' lives. Thus, state-subsidized, high-quality child care remains a critical policy issue for facilitating women's employment and economic well-being, just as Esping-Andersen now recognizes with his child-centred social investment strategy. By no means should the analysis in the chapter be interpreted as lending support for the assumption, prevalent in liberal welfare regimes, that care for children under age six is predominantly a private responsibility of the parents who birth or raise them.

Rather, at issue in the first question is the broader project of work-family balance that policy makers must grapple with as they address the challenges that citizens face in terms of synchronizing their care and work responsibilities and aspirations throughout the life course. I will argue in Chapter 7 that, in addition to universal child care, this balance depends on the institutionalization of citizenry entitlements to flexible, generously paid care benefits that provide individuals with subsidized time to attend to their child, elder, and other dependent care interests and obligations. The challenge is to determine how much time should, and can, be subsidized. Similarly, labour standards regulating hours of paid work have a role to play in promoting work-family balance in liberal welfare regimes. The alignment of social inclusion with time for kin caregiving favours public policy strategies that reduce standard full-time workweeks and workyears by inducing citizens to take future productivity gains in the form of less paid worktime.

The issue of time for informal care poses particularly challenging public policy issues in terms of single parents, the large majority of whom are women. Cross-nationally there is a trend toward obliging single mothers to pursue paid work despite the presence of young children (Knijn 1994; Knijn and Kremer 1997; Roberts 1995b, 199). We have seen that British Columbia offers one recent example now that legislation requires "employable" lone parents to seek work when their youngest child turns three, down from age seven.

Scholars like Knijn (1994), who defend a right to time for care, and Mink (2002), who is concerned that this right is denied, particularly among poor racial minority women, approach this policy trend with trepidation. Knijn (1994, 103), for instance, maintains that "women should be allowed to claim the right to an income from [caring for children]. Women who take care of children during the years that other citizens are making their way in the labor force are handicapping themselves in terms of their career ambitions, but I do not think that this implies that every mother should pursue a career, with all the troubles of organizing personal life that it entails."

There is much reason to be cautious about the position defended by Knijn and Mink, however. It simply is not reasonable to posit that a choice *not* to engage in paid work so long as children live at home is a realistic path to social inclusion (see also Orloff 1997, 193-94). The opportunity costs in terms of forgone income and economic security are too great, particularly in societies that valorize a paid work ethic. Once again the issue is: How much time for domestic care does social inclusion require? On this topic, further work is needed to determine whether the BC and other governments allow single parents to enjoy sufficient time to care.

The second policy question – how do we embrace time for domestic care as a necessary condition for social inclusion without further entrenching patriarchy? – speaks to the gender division of labour that cuts across ethnocultural groups. Shachar (2000, 203), for instance, observes that women's "crucial cultural roles have traditionally been expressed in the realm of the family, through adherence to a set of gender-biased norms and practices which often subordinate women."

Although Shachar alerts us to the potential tension between accommodating cultural diversity through domestic care and showing due concern for female autonomy (Shachar 2000, 201; Saharso 2000), much African American feminist literature rejects the notion that challenging intragroup oppression of women, including "the exploitative aspects of black women's labor in their homes," threatens to derail efforts to secure the survival of ethnocultural identity (Roberts 1995b, 205). "The question of women doing more than their fair share of [caregiving] work for individual and community development," Collins (1994, 50) argues, "merits open debate." This debate has yet to develop fully, Roberts (1995a, 245) believes, since some women of colour "remain silent about sexism in [their] communities" out of "fear that [they] will be charged with betraying" the community's "common interests as a people" in the struggle against racism. However, in the absence of such debate, any celebration of "heroic African American mothers" whose care is integral to the retention of group identity amounts to "a cruel form of romanticism" that diverts attention from the sexism historically sanctioned as part of the collective struggle against racism (Roberts 1995b, 205).

The need to challenge cross-cultural practices that permit men's privileged irresponsibility for care is the subject of the next chapter. Like Cass (1994, 114-15), who argues that a "democratic conception of citizenship" should "be based unequivocally on the understanding that men cannot be accorded full citizenship if they do not fulfill their responsibilities for care-giving work," I favour dramatic reform of public policy to institutionalize care as an obligation of citizenship that equally binds men and women.

Reprioritizing time for domestic care is not just about minimizing the harm that many men inflict on women as a result of their irresponsibility for care. Although the Collins-inspired literature focuses on mother-work, an important implication of the finding that social inclusion comprises time for domesticity and care is that many successful male breadwinners also do not enjoy full social inclusion; they are marginalized from an important sphere of affectivity, which leaves some care ambitions unfulfilled or even undiscovered. For instance, in a recent longitudinal, qualitative study of first-time fathers, Barclay and Lupton (1999, 1019) report that

> nearly all our participants found fatherhood, in the beginning at least, to be disappointing and frustrating. Most of the group expected to be

more involved than they actually were. Clearly the "absent father" the men said they had experienced with their own father as children was no longer acceptable to this generation of men, but many were replicating this through force of circumstance rather than choice ...

A most remarkable feature of the experiences of this group of first-time fathers is how most remained on the fringes of parenthood for the first 6 months [the duration of the study]. The emotional rewards for new fathers appeared to be in proportion to the amount of time and energy they expended in intimate contact with the child. Only a minority of participants did not want to provide this care, but most men found it difficult to find the time away from paid employment to develop the skills they required to do so adequately.

The theme of male exclusion from family spaces is now receiving some attention abroad, particularly in the Netherlands and Sweden. The Dutch Ministry of Social Affairs has launched an educational media campaign to re-image masculinity and fatherhood. It presents a young boy sitting at a dining room table with his father and siblings. When his mother enters the room, the boy alludes to the father's limited involvement in family life by asking, "Who is this man who cuts the meat every Sunday?" (Knijn and Selten 2002, 168). The Swedish government employs the image of the "velour papa" for the similar purpose of challenging masculine norms, famously portraying a celebrity weightlifter holding a small infant in his arms (Bergman and Hobson 2002, 107). In light of the arguments in this chapter, there is need for Canada and other liberal welfare regimes to engage in a comparable project of redefining cultural metaphors of masculinity and fatherhood so that women and men alike can increasingly embrace time for informal care and the social belonging that is available among family and fictive kin.

7
Care*fair*

The political shift that rebalances rights talk with renewed emphasis on social obligations is incomplete and inadequate whenever duty discourses do not engage with care responsibilities, especially men's relative neglect of caregiving regardless of their class and ethnic affiliation (Coltrane 1996; Kamo and Cohen 1998). The Pateman literature reveals that men's free riding on female care inflicts harm on diverse groups of women, largely by impeding their equal participation in social, political, and economic spaces outside of the domestic sphere and by undermining their financial security. The Collins literature, in contrast, provides reason to worry that the irresponsibility for care from which many men benefit in the market is nonetheless self-injurious. If private time for domestic care is necessary for social inclusion, then the cultural, public policy, and company-level expectations for ideal employees, which prescribe extensive hours in the paid labour market, risk marginalizing the most economically successful men and women from an important sphere of affectivity. The same risk is also encountered by citizens who suffer limited earnings potential because financial need forces them to labour long hours in low-wage work at the expense of private time in the web of domestic relations that is often foundational to social belonging.

In this chapter I propose the concept of care*fair* to remedy the short-comings in neoliberal, third way, communitarian, and social conservative invocations of citizenship duties. Care*fair* engages with the essential ambivalence to connection that Gilligan (1987, 32) observes in her discussion of the ethics of care and justice. The concept acknowledges that care labour is often a source of disadvantage for diverse groups of women because many men with whom they share group membership are not culturally, politically, or economically expected to perform a fair share of care work. The appropriate response to this source of inequality, however, is not to help all citizens minimize the contribution they make to the social product through caregiving, as Esping-Andersen's vision of the social investment state would have it. Rather, the solution rests in embracing private time for caregiving as a constitutive element of full social membership. Since care work is critical for social reproduction, it is reasonable for the public to expect all citizens to make a minimum contribution to society's care needs as a condition of benefiting from the mutual advantages made possible by community collaboration. Consistent with the Collins-inspired literature, the care*fair* concept also recognizes that private time for domestic care is intrinsically valuable as a source of pleasure, protection, fulfillment, and affirmation. A care*fair* agenda would, therefore, institutionalize through social policy new opportunities for citizens to enjoy time in their domestic spaces that would not compromise their financial security or that of their dependants.

Care*fair* is an analogue to workfare and other active labour market measures. Through workfare, governments employ the power of public policy to compel citizens to fulfill their employment duties as a condition of receipt of social assistance. The care*fair* idea implores governments to demonstrate a comparable level of concern to address the morally hazardous dynamics that inhere in the gender division of care. The aim is to redesign public policy in order to change the system of societal incentives in which men make decisions about how much time to allocate between employment and caregiving. Under care*fair*, the incentive structure would be reorganized to urge men to assume a more equitable share of the informal care work that is just as essential to social (re)production as is market participation.

As an analogue to workfare, care*fair* does not lend intellectual support to any specific active labour market policy that exists cross-nationally. Nor does it deny the punitive character of workfare in some North American jurisdictions, including the province of British Columbia (for example, Klein and Long 2003). Instead, the concept affirms the theoretical defence of welfare contractualism that S. White (2000) offers. Care*fair* embraces the position that social rights imply an unconditional entitlement of reasonable access to some social good, where "reasonable access" connotes that a citizen can attain the good without unreasonable effort. This understanding of entitlement allows us to retain the enormous value of social rights to which Marshall and Rawls point, while compensating for the risks to civic-mindedness that social liberalism permits because it underemphasizes the question of social duties. Care*fair* thus accepts in principle a policy that renders receipt of social benefits conditional on the discharge of social duties so long as the conditions for fair reciprocity exist within the community. The care*fair* concept qualifies White's arguments, however, by insisting that caregiving factors in what counts as a duty, as well as what counts as a reasonable contribution to the social product.

It is necessary to establish a better equilibrium between social rights and obligations in order to address "the patriarchal dividend," to borrow a phrase from Connell (1995, 79), from which all men benefit as a result of the cultural subordination of women. The habit of free riding on female care permitted half the population is a much more significant case of moral hazard than is the risk that welfare benefits may erode the motivation to engage in paid work of a relatively small percentage of citizens on social assistance. The legacy of patriarchy includes a diverse range of cultural, political, and economic incentives that induce men to behave in socially non-optimal ways by performing less caregiving than they could in the absence of the gender division of care. As Taylor-Goodby (1991, 202-3) notes, many state welfare systems in turn "act as a transmission mechanism" for these inequalities that originate elsewhere. Whenever social policy does not explicitly challenge the gender division of labour, it risks becoming implicated in, and contributing to, the pattern of incentives that induce many men to evade care work. In such instances, the welfare state emerges as "an apparatus of moral hazard" in respect of the critical area of social life that the numerous informal systems of domestic care provision represent. Three notable Canadian examples illustrate the point: employment leave policies, employment standards regulating full-time hours, and child care.

Moral Hazard Apparatus 1: Employment Leave
Research consistently confirms that the birth of a child sets in motion a series of normative expectations and economic incentives that propel many heterosexual couples to approximate patriarchal patterns in the division of labour. Spouses become more traditional in their care, housework, and employment decisions upon the onset of parenthood, with the most significant changes occurring in women's routines. In particular, the total amount of work that new mothers perform increases disproportionately compared to new fathers, although relatively little of this extra work is in paid employment (for a review of this literature, see Sanchez and Thomson 1997).

Decisions by spousal units to reduce the mother's paid work, particularly following a parental leave period, have long-term consequences for the division of care (Coltrane 1996, 71). Zvonkovic et al. (1996, 99) observe that, "when a couple makes a work-family decision that, to some extent, limits or restricts the wife's paid work, even if this decision is viewed as temporary and is made for reasons other than conformity to traditional attitudes, the enactment of this decision can serve to sweep the couple along a sea of traditional cultural attitudes and gender work force realities."

Parenthood often crystallizes the gender division of labour because the person who limits attachment to the paid workforce to nurture an infant, typically the female partner, becomes especially knowledgeable and skilled in rearing the child by virtue of her regular, daily caring experiences. In contrast, reduced female earnings often motivate a male spouse to increase employment hours to compensate for the loss of household income. His stronger attachment to the labour market limits the time available to acquire familiarity and expertise in caring for his children when they are very young. The result, Lupton and Barclay (1997, 148) report, is that "it is all too easy for men to lag behind their female partner in developing the skills of caring for their children, even when the men may strongly wish to do so, and it can be difficult for them to make up for the lost ground."

Maternity and parental leave policy in Canada exacerbate this dynamic, despite recent improvements to the leave benefit system. In 2001 the Canadian federal government introduced new provisions that extended the combined maternity/parental leave benefit period available through Employment Insurance (EI) from roughly six months to fifty weeks.[1] The increased benefit period cost the government $1 billion annually in 2003, raising the annual expenditure on leave to $2.4 billion in that year (Chief Actuary 2001, 9-13). Leave benefits must be used in the child's first year. Fifteen weeks of the leave period are defined as maternity leave, for which only biological mothers are eligible. The remaining thirty-five weeks are characterized as parental leave and may be taken by the mother or father (biological or adopted), or shared by both. The value of maternity/parental leave benefits is income contingent, calculated at a rate of 55 percent of the recipient's earnings up to a maximum benefit of $413 a week. Access to supplementary employer-sponsored leave benefits is rare in Canada. Just one in five mothers on leave in 2001 reported additional leave remuneration above what is provided through EI (K. Marshall 2003, 6).

The value of leave benefits in Canada presently constitutes a barrier to male participation in the program. The benefit system generates financial incentives for the lower earner in a heterosexual couple to take the leave, since a couple maximizes household income by deciding not to incur the minimum 45 percent reduction from the higher earner's salary. Given the persistent gender earnings gap, the lower earner is more often the mother. Together, the structural incentive implicit in the policy and the gender earnings differential help to explain why just 2 percent of parental leave benefit recipients in Canada were fathers prior to the extension of the benefit period in 2001 (Statistics Canada 2000, 109). Since the policy change, there has been a notable increase in the number of Canadian men taking advantage of leave benefits. However, fathers still represented just 7 percent of benefit recipients in the first year, and only 11 percent in the second year (Canada Employment Insurance Commission 2003, 18). Men also stay on leave for a much shorter period. The median claim period for men in 2001-2 was fifteen weeks, compared to thirty weeks for women (ibid.).

Moral Hazard Apparatus 2: Employment Standards
Regulating Full-Time Work
In the first decades following the Second World War, policy makers invoked the concept of a family wage that would provide sufficient income for a male breadwinner to support his dependent wife and children (Orloff 1993, 319; Pateman 1989, 189; Slaughter 1995, 78). While only the most powerful unions in Canada were generally successful in this era in achieving levels of remuneration sufficient to maintain an entire family (Luxton and Reiter 1997, 200), the discourse reflected policy assumptions that presumed a functional division between breadwinner and caregiver. The family wage concept assumed that the primary earner in a household would be relatively unencumbered by familial or other responsibilities that might limit his flexibility to respond to employer needs.

Significant labour force restructuring over the past three decades resulted in revised labour patterns that re-entrenched this functional division between primary earner and care provider, despite the rapid increase in the number of women in the labour force. The division remains strong because the so-called standard workweek has become less common in the last three decades as the distribution of paid work hours among Canadians in the labour market polarized. The proportion of people working thirty-five to forty hours per week declined, with corresponding increases in the share of people working both short and long workweeks. Three Canadian studies confirm this trend (Hall 1999; Morissette, Myles, and Picot 1995; Sheridan, Sunter, and Diverty 1996). While figures from the studies differ for methodological reasons, all three find that the proportion of people working standard weekly hours has dropped by roughly 10 percent since 1975. The study by Hall (1999,

30) indicates that the "standard" week ceased to be the norm for the majority of Canadians by 1980; she reports that as few as 41 percent of workers laboured thirty-five to forty hours per week by the end of the 1990s.

Labour patterns among all workers indicate that the shift toward short workweeks has been more pronounced than the shift toward longer hours (Hall 1999; Sheridan, Sunter, and Diverty 1996). This trend reflects the dramatic increase in the number of women in the labour force and the fact that women are much more likely than men to work part-time hours. But when data are broken down by gender, the most significant proportional gain for both female and male workers was in positions in which they worked more than forty weekly hours (Morissette, Myles, and Picot 1995, 37). Between 1976 and 1995, the share of men who usually worked long hours increased by more than five percentage points (from 19.0 percent to 24.3 percent), versus a three-point increase in short weeks (from 3.9 percent to 7.1 percent). During the same period, the share of women who usually put in long workweeks rose nearly three percentage points (from 5.8 percent to 8.6 percent), whereas the percentage usually working short weeks rose slightly less at just over two points (from 27.7 percent to 30.1 percent) (Sheridan, Sunter, and Diverty 1996, C12).

The polarization in working time since 1976 converged with job characteristics relating to earnings, education, industrial sector, and age, with the result that the redistribution of paid work powered a growing gap between a core and a contingent labour force. Long workweeks grew more common for high-wage earners, the university educated, managers, professionals, and blue-collar workers in typically male industries, such as processing, machining, fabricating, construction, and transport operations, where paid overtime opportunities are relatively common (Sheridan, Sunter, and Diverty 1996, C19-C20; Duchesne 1997). Conversely, the growth in short workweeks was more concentrated in the predominantly female service sector, especially among low-wage workers, persons with no post-secondary certificate, women over fifty-five, and workers ages fifteen to twenty-four who were no longer in school (Morissette, Myles, and Picot 1995, 38; Sheridan, Sunter, and Diverty 1996, C10-C14).

The convergence of worker characteristics with the polarization of worktime signals that employers in many industries rely increasingly on a core of relatively well-paid, educated, and experienced workers for longer hours (Morissette, Myles, and Picot 1995, 38; Sheridan,

Sunter, and Diverty 1996, C26). The effect of this labour usage reform is to further entrench the norm of the ideal worker as someone
unencumbered by responsibilities that limit one's willingness to commit to the job to the degree demanded by an employer. Occupations
that pay well and/or grant substantial responsibility give employees less
time to spend on non-paid work aspirations and needs, including
caregiving, than was the case in the mid-1970s.

The polarization of paid worktime provides little reason to believe
that the functional division of responsibilities between ideal worker and
unpaid caregiver is blurring, despite the marked increase in the share of
mothers of young children in the labour force. Unless an ideal employee
chooses to remain childless, as more Canadians are doing (Duxbury
and Higgins 2003), someone else must assume responsibility for her or
his children in order to free this employee to be a member of the core
staff. Whoever assumes this unpaid responsibility disqualifies herself or
himself from the category of ideal worker and is, therefore, far more
likely to work at the margins of the market if she or he endeavours to
maintain some attachment to the labour force. At the margins, economic sustainability is increasingly difficult to achieve as hours, pay,
and benefits decline. The polarization of paid worktime witnessed in
Canada therefore reinforces the risk of economic dependence – on either
an ideal worker or the state – for anyone who takes on (or wishes to take
on) a significant role providing unpaid care, even though that person is
also far more likely to be in the labour force today than she or he would
have been thirty years ago.

Recent changes to employment standards, which fall under provincial jurisdiction in Canada, are reinforcing the functional division between principal earner and caregiver. In 2000, Ontario blazed new ground
on the path toward enabling employers to rely on core workers well
beyond the forty-hour weekly norm. Legislation allows firms to design
work-hour arrangements that permit employees to work as many as
180 hours in a three-week period (averaging sixty hours per week). Ontario employees can refuse work only after labouring forty-eight hours
in one week, and they are due overtime compensation only after forty-
four hours (Government of Ontario 2000).

The government in British Columbia has followed a comparable path.
Additional flexibility was initially assigned the high-tech sector in 1999,
when policy changes altogether exempted high-tech professionals from
Parts 4 and 5 of the provincial Employment Standards Act (ESA), which
regulate hours of work, overtime, and statutory holidays. In 2002 the

government extended greater flexibility to the entire labour market by introducing the concept of "averaging agreements" to the ESA (s. 37). Similar to those in Ontario, these agreements permit managers to schedule employees for hours outside the standard eight-hour day and forty-hour week by calculating average employment time over a period of up to four weeks. This policy change allows employees to work as many as twelve hours in a single day without being paid overtime, so long as total hours over the multiple-week period do not exceed an average of forty hours in seven days.

Policy that extends the number of weekly hours expected of ideal employees reinforces systemic barriers to successful labour force participation among people with significant unpaid care obligations and aspirations. The consequences for single parents burdened with the challenge of balancing earning and caring on their own may be particularly adverse, since they have the least flexibility to approximate this ideal employee norm, especially in the absence of affordable, quality child care. The longer hours required of core employees also increases the likelihood that heterosexual couples will approximate the primary breadwinner/primary caregiver family model, which we have seen remains the norm within a majority of households that are home to a child under twelve.

Moral Hazard Apparatus 3: Child Care Policy

Extensive historical, policy, and theoretical literatures reveal that child care responsibilities structure labour market opportunities for women very differently than for men cross-nationally (for example, Sainsbury 1994). Econometric studies attempt to quantify the negative influence that child care costs exert on female labour supply. Two Canadian studies draw similar conclusions. Powell (1997) and Cleveland, Gunderson, and Hyatt (1996) find that a 10 percent increase in the expected price of child care correlates with reductions in the probability that a mother will engage in paid work of 3.8 and 3.9 percent respectively. These Canadian findings fall in the middle range of US results (for example, Kimmel 1998; Ribar 1995). Powell further suggests that a 10 percent increase in child care costs corresponds with a 3.2 percent decrease in the number of paid hours that mothers work. Cleveland, Gunderson, and Hyatt (1996) add that a 10 percent rise in child care fees will result in an 11 percent reduction in the probability that the mother will purchase care arrangements, with the result that care work is shifted to unpaid settings. A shift from formal arrangements for which a fee is paid to more informal care contexts further weakens the labour market ties of people (almost always women) who agree to provide care at no, or very reduced, cost.

These econometric data confirm that welfare state policy regarding child care, also a provincial responsibility in Canada, is significantly implicated in the rate at which women access employment and the resulting gender division of labour. In the international arena, Canada is weak in terms of child care. In a comparison of child benefit packages in twenty-two of the most prosperous countries, Bradshaw and Finch (2002, Table 5.1) find that Canada ranks last in terms of the share of three- and four-year-olds in licensed child care or education. Just 23 percent of Canadian children in this age category use such services, nineteen percentage points below Britain, the country ranked twenty-first. By contrast, in France all three- and four-year-olds are in child care or education, as are over 90 percent of children in that age group in Denmark, the Netherlands, New Zealand, and Spain.

Policy in the province of British Columbia contributes to Canada's status as an international laggard vis-à-vis child care. As of 2001, there were enough regulated child care spaces in the province for only 12 percent of children from birth to age twelve. The provincial government allocates just $274 per year per child under thirteen for regulated child care (Childcare Resource and Research Unit 2002, Tables 30 and 34a). This *annual* public expenditure is considerably less than the average cost of *monthly* fees for regulated care in the province, which range from $494 to $705 depending on the care context and child's age (Forer and Hunter 2001).

The province recently had a plan in place to address more aggressively the barrier that child care costs pose for women's employment. In the final year of its mandate, the New Democratic Party (NDP) government introduced the Child Care BC Act (SBC 2001, c. 4). The act established a plan to subsidize the cost of child care for all children regardless of parental income by creating a new expenditure delivery mechanism, the Funding Assistance Program (FAP). FAP was designed to inject $353 million in new operating funding for licensed centre-based or "group" child care services, as well as for "family child care" programs run by self-employed women out of their own residences. Providers were eligible to receive FAP on the condition that they limit fees to a maximum of $14 for full day care and $7 for before- and after-school services.

The act set a four-year timeline to phase in the additional funds. However, the NDP implemented only the first phase before its electoral defeat, entering into contracts with licensed out-of-school programs to subsidize 17,000 spaces at a cost of $30 million annually. Following its election to office in 2001, the new Liberal government amended the Child Care BC Act, eliminating sections that committed the government to universally reducing the cost of care (Miscellaneous Statutes Amendment Act, SBC 2001, c. 32). In place of new expenditures, the government further reduced the provincial child care budget by roughly $50 million annually (Kershaw 2004).

In light of the above econometric research, the Liberal government's decision to rescind the universal child care system abandons the substantial positive consequences for women's employment that the reduction of daily fees for full day care to $14 would have generated and, thus, accepts the status quo gender division of labour. This maximum daily charge would have reduced the mean provincial fee for licensed care by between 40 and 58 percent, depending on the care setting and the child's age. Evidence suggests that such a reduction would have correlated with a 15 to 22 percent increase in the probability that mothers would have accepted paid work.

Restructuring the Context of Choice

These three examples of moral hazard that implicate state policy illuminate how the employment decisions that many fathers make, regardless of their conscious intentions, generate what economists define as negative externalities. When fathers accept long hours of employment following the birth of a child, they enter into contracts to exchange their labour for remuneration. But the full range of costs associated with the exchange is not borne exclusively by the contractor and contractee. Given the legacy of patriarchy, costs are also imposed on diverse groups of women, who are external to the contract, by virtue of the fact that their care labour, whether for no or modest pay, will likely be required to free fathers to work long hours in the market.

The remedy to this problem requires recognition that, although we make choices, we do not do so in contexts of our own choosing. Patriarchy means that men from diverse class and ethnic groups inherit a social structure that induces them to free ride on the reproductive work of others. If gender equality is a social priority, it is necessary to reform the context of choice that men inherit. This is the objective of care*fair*. It advocates policy change to revise normative and financial incentives to which men respond so that the incentives are more likely to entice men to embrace a greater share of informal caregiving.

The underlying objective of care*fair* is the same one that informs Fraser's universal caregiver model: to induce far more men to modify their behaviour and attitudes so that they act more like most contemporary women, who perform primary care work in addition to employment and other citizenry ambitions and responsibilities. A primary change implied by this objective is a revamped ideal worker norm to reflect the view that the social citizen is neither wholly a labour force participant nor only an unpaid caregiver, but a citizen who interweaves both roles. This conceptual shift would extend to all men the caregiver half of the postwar breadwinner/caregiver model, just as the breadwinner role has been extended (at least ideologically) to women through pay and employment equity legislation.

If realized, one consequence of care*fair* would be a significant share of women participating in the marketplace and other important areas of public life more than they do at present. But it is imperative to recognize that the universal caregiver model, at least as I employ it, does not set as a goal the minimization of domestic time, especially when men's and women's care work is under consideration collectively. Instead, this model takes for granted that time for care in one's web of domestic relations is a critical element of full social membership that needs to be preserved, if not enhanced, as discussed in the previous chapter. Thus, a care*fair* policy platform does not just strive for greater sharing of employment and caring between the sexes; it also aims to institutionalize policy that will provide all citizens with sufficient time for domestic care without compromising individual or familial financial security.

The care*fair* focus on public policy does not imply that the state is the sole cause of the patriarchal division of care. The second shift falls overwhelmingly to women for many interlocking reasons (for example, Olson 2002). Still, insofar as government programs and regulatory measures are implicated as apparatuses of moral hazard, policy reform represents one accessible opportunity to begin redefining the cultural context in which men and women make decisions between employment and caring. The rest of the chapter concentrates on the three policy envelopes already considered. I propose care*fair* reforms for leave benefits, employment standards regulating full-time work, and child care funding. While these three policy areas are significant engines of moral hazard, they are not alone. The tax system is also a pervasive policy mechanism that shapes the social context in which individual choices are embedded. Elsewhere I have identified problems with Canada's income tax treatment of caregiving and dependency and proposed policy solutions (Kershaw 2002).

Care*fair* Reform 1: Paid Worktime Reductions over the Life Course
A welfare regime premised on the assumption that the social citizen is a
worker and caregiver must minimize the functional division of responsibilities between the two roles. This division is weakened only if institutional arrangements are reorganized to allow citizens' legitimate family
ambitions and responsibilities to become more compatible with the paid
work practices of core staff. Institutional change will require redefinition of labour market norms regulating employment hours to reduce the
time that ideal workers are expected to commit to their jobs, particularly
during life-course stages when unpaid careloads are especially acute.

Maternity and parental leave benefits represent one obvious place to
redefine full-time employment expectations over the life course. These
benefits subsidize and have potential to normalize extended periods of
labour market withdrawal for citizens when careloads increase. Numerous changes to the Canadian federal leave system are necessary to achieve
this end, including the following five reforms.

1   The leave system should be removed from Employment Insurance
    (EI) administrative mechanisms and financed through general tax
    revenue to which the self-employed contribute.
2   The value of benefits should be increased on two fronts: the level of
    remuneration should be calculated as 80 percent of previous income,
    and the maximum monthly benefit should plateau at annual incomes
    of $50,000, rather than the present $39,000 limit.
3   While the value of benefits should remain contingent on income,
    eligibility conditions should be loosened to capture a greater share
    of the population employed part-time. The parental benefit system
    would ideally encompass a minimum flat-rate benefit even for par-
    ents who do not meet employment eligibility criteria. The mini-
    mum benefit would recognize the social value of quality early
    childhood development experiences provided by parents during a
    child's early years.
4   The number of months of benefits available to a household should
    be extended. A substantial portion of the time should be reserved
    exclusively for fathers, with appropriate exceptions for single, di-
    vorced, and lesbian parents. When fathers do not make use of this
    reserved time, the leave system should not permit the benefits to be
    transferred to the mother, and the reserved time should be deducted
    from the total benefit period available to the family.
5   Take-up of maternity and parental leave benefits should be linked
    with eligibility for the Canada and Quebec Pension Plans (C/QPP)

so that every month on leave reduces the total amount of employment time one must bank before being eligible for a full C/QPP.

The first reform proposal reflects the need to expand eligibility for
maternity and parental leave benefits. In 2001, 39 percent of mothers
with newborns did not receive birth-related benefits. Of these women,
23 percent went without benefits because they were not employed before the birth of the child; another 12 percent were paid workers who
were not eligible for benefits due to their insufficient employment history or because they simply did not apply; and 5 percent received no
leave benefits because they were self-employed and, therefore, ineligible for EI benefits of any kind, including maternity and parental leave
(K. Marshall 2003, 6).

These data indicate a sizable share of part-time workers continues to
pay EI premiums without the opportunity to cash in on leave benefits,
while self-employed workers remain ineligible regardless of their attachment to the labour market. The latter is particularly worrisome given
that the self-employed are a growing segment of the labour force, representing nearly one in every five workers. The exclusion of self-employed
citizens from the leave system also contributes to the less frequent participation of fathers in the program since men represent roughly two-
thirds of the self-employed. This exclusionary character of the current
system could be addressed by amending eligibility so that any citizen
with annual earnings of $2,000 or more would be entitled to benefits,
thereby including most part-time and self-employed individuals. An
alternative policy option would see the introduction of a minimum
benefit of $100 per month (indexed to inflation) that would render the
leave benefit program universal. This alternative would parallel policy
in Sweden and Norway, where a flat-rate benefit is available for parents
with limited or no labour force attachment who do not qualify for parental leave benefits based on their previous earnings (Baker 1995, 176;
European Industrial Relations Review 2001a, 18). In either case, the
changes would require that Canada detach the leave benefit system from
EI in favour of funding the program from general revenue to ensure
that self-employed citizens receive benefits from a pool of public revenue to which they contribute.

In addition to increasing eligibility, it is necessary to enrich the value
of parental leave benefits in order to increase the range of caregiving
options genuinely available to low-income and single parents. Raising
benefit levels from 55 to 80 percent of earnings would render the choice
of providing child care personally more feasible because it is more afford-

able. The minimum 45 percent drop in income mandated by the present system means that expectant mothers must earn incomes at the maximum insurable level – roughly $750 per week – if they are to receive a benefit income equal to the low-income cut-off for a two-person family residing in Canada's largest cities (approximately $415 a week). By contrast, the average weekly value of maternity benefits received by Canadian mothers is $277 (Statistics Canada 1999b). This level of income is not enough for many poor and single parents given that the costs associated with a newborn typically raise private expenditures.

Since immigrant women, women of colour, Aboriginal women, and women with disabilities are disproportionately likely to earn incomes that yield very low benefit levels (Statistics Canada 2000, Chapters 9 to 11), Iyer (1997, 171) observes that the "typical recipient of the benefit emerges as a white, middle-class, female employee, over 25, with either a higher than average income, or more likely, partnered with someone else who is the primary income earner." Thus, the structure of the present benefit system means there is a group of women who pay employment insurance premiums despite being disqualified from taking advantage of maternity leave because they cannot afford the drop in earnings that the system entails. The implication is that the premiums of less economically advantaged women "subsidize the reproductive activities of more economically privileged women" (176). This scenario will only be minimized if the value of leave benefits is increased to 80 percent or more of insurable earnings, since low-wage or single women are more likely to be able to afford a 20 percent reduction in income than a 45 percent cut following the birth of a child.

While care*fair* recommends a minimum maternity/parental leave benefit in recognition of the social value of childrearing, the system should retain the current logic, which links benefit levels to previous earnings. This logic is important because the timing of reproductive decisions along the life course influences the gender division of labour. Coltrane (1996, 126-33) reports that heterosexual spousal units which share household work most equally tend to delay childbearing until at least their late twenties or early thirties. Delaying the transition to parenthood increases the likelihood that women will continue employment following the birth of a child, because a period of childlessness gives women time to develop strong employment-related identities (Drolet 2002b). Postponing parenthood also appears to help men avoid some of the financial and time constraints that early-birth fathers face when endeavouring to forge simultaneously employment and fatherhood identities. In keeping with this research, a leave system that calculates benefits on the basis of previous earnings is advantageous because it represents a structural incentive for parents to delay childrearing until they develop stronger labour market attachments that yield more valuable benefits.

Beyond the life-course timing of parenthood, research also shows that the point at which a father involves himself in primary child care has long-term consequences for the man's participation in childrearing and other household work. Coltrane (1996, 82-83) reports that heterosexual couples who generally share most responsibility for care and domestic labour tend to involve the father in routine child care from early infancy. Similarly, research from Canada and Sweden indicates that men who take advantage of parental leave tend to spend more time childrearing throughout their children's lives (Baker 1997, 66). This research provides further reason to revamp and enrich maternity/parental leave entitlements in Canada to counter the structural barrier that limited benefit rates, in combination with the gender earnings gap, pose to leave participation among fathers. The structural barrier is minimized the more that policy reduces the financial loss families incur when the higher earner withdraws from the labour force. A leave system that remunerates 80, rather than 55, percent of previous earnings up to a maximum annual salary of $50,000, rather than $39,000, would represent significant progress on this front. In Sweden, where remuneration rates are 80 percent of previous income, data indicate that a bare majority of fathers now participate in the leave program (O'Hara 1998, 16-17). This figure far exceeds paternal participation in Canada, which stands at 11 percent as of 2001 (Canada Employment Insurance Commission 2003, 18).

Mitigating the legacy of patriarchy will require more than increased benefit rates, however. The two countries that stand out in terms of the share of fathers who take some parental leave are Norway and Sweden. Norway appears especially exceptional in that roughly 70 percent of fathers take some leave (Leira 1998, 370-71; K. Marshall 2003, 10). What is unique about these countries is that both reserve some leave time exclusively for new fathers. In 1993 Norway led the way on this front by reserving four weeks of leave. If a father does not make use of this time, it cannot be transferred to the mother and is deducted from the overall benefit (European Industrial Relations Review 2001a, 18). The Swedish government followed suit in 1995, also reserving thirty days of leave for fathers (2001b, 14-15).

The results of the Swedish experience suggest the importance of being aggressive with daddy leave policy. The introduction of the one daddy month in 1995 saw the share of male parental leave recipients in Sweden rise 2.6 percentage points (from 28.5 to 31.1 percent) by 1996, an increase that surpassed that of the previous four years combined. The accelerated pace of male participation continued throughout the rest of the decade, so that 37.7 percent of benefit recipients were fathers as of 2000. However, Swedish men still only use 12.4 percent of the days for which a parental allowance is paid by the state, up from 9.2 percent in 1995 and 7.7 percent at the beginning of the decade.[2] In response to the increased (albeit still small) share of days that men take, the Swedish government acknowledged that reserving one month remains too little an incentive to challenge gendered expectations in households and the market. The solution the government has followed is to extend the period of leave reserved exclusively for fathers to two months. No data documenting the impact of this policy change on male behavioural patterns are yet available.

Building on the Swedish experience, a commitment to care*fair* would see the Canadian federal government require fathers in two-parent families (making appropriate exceptions for single, divorced, and lesbian parents) to use at least two, and ideally four, months of the fifty-week leave period. If the value of leave benefits is enriched to 80 percent of previous earnings, the four-month requirement would constitute a significant incentive for men to involve themselves early in primary child care. Econometric research is required to determine the rate at which men in Canada can be expected to respond to daddy months by taking some or all of the time.

Some may worry that reserving several months of the existing leave period for fathers risks penalizing women (through loss of benefits to which they are currently eligible) who reside with male partners unwilling to take advantage of the daddy months. The care*fair* reform would minimize this risk because it proposes to increase benefit levels from 55 to 80 percent of previous income, representing a 45 percent increase in the value of leave benefits. As a result of the proposed changes, a woman could, therefore, replace in 8 months the value of forgone earnings that she receives in 11.6 months under the current system. The mother would be free to allocate the financial assistance over a fifty-week period and enjoy the same length of leave at roughly the same benefit rate that is currently available under EI. Although it may seem unfair (particularly for mothers) that heterosexual households with fathers who avoid caregiving will receive fewer months of leave, social policy that does not alter the patriarchal division of care also imposes costs on women that are unjust. These costs manifest themselves in far broader social ills, including the gender earnings gap, feminization of poverty, and women's under-representation in political spheres.

The risk to women with resistant spouses could be minimized entirely by extending the total duration of leave benefits to accommodate the daddy months, rather than setting aside benefits for men from within the time currently available to households. Recent Canadian experience affirms the value of extending the benefit period if undercutting patriarchy is a priority. Pérusse (2003, 14) reports a fivefold increase in the number of fathers who took leave one year after the benefit period was extended by six months, compared to the number who took leave the year before the policy change. The extended leave period means that new mothers can now share leave benefits with spouses without sacrificing time off in the final weeks of the last trimester, when pregnancy is often a physical ordeal. Longer leaves would facilitate more male participation in the program without limiting the time away from work that allows new mothers to breastfeed. Research by Lupton and Barclay (1997, 138) indicates that breastfeeding is a factor that tends to limit men's role in early childrearing, even among fathers who express a strong desire to involve themselves intimately in the care of their newborns.

The limited share of leave time that fathers take in Sweden provides reason to remain skeptical that the reservation of benefits exclusively for fathers will trigger an immediate refashioning of the gender order in Canada. A number of scholars who examine parental leave among Swedish parents point to the significance of gender symbolism in explaining the still-modest response to daddy months by men (for example, Bergman and Hobson 2002; Brandth and Kvande 1998). Højgaard (1997, 258), for instance, argues that a father's decision to care actively for (not just about) his newborn "challenges a very basic symbolic meaning of masculinity as it involves work performance." The decision also runs contrary to other "structural elements of the symbolic order of gender such as the gendering of the economy, the cultural prescriptions of 'good' mothering, and expert advice on child raising" (251). Højgaard suggests that the resulting symbolic discord between male employment and active caregiving is one "reason that men do not take full advantage of the possibilities of ameliorating the contradictions between work and family that are, albeit ambiguously, offered by the work place culture and by welfare state policies" (258). Symbolic coding of masculinity and parental leave means that the task of obliging men to fulfill a fair share of care must first clash with the very cultural norms that are the product and self-preservation of patriarchy. As Højgaard puts it, parental leave will become a practicable entitlement of fathers "only on certain conditions" (251). It is a right that is ultimately "dependent on the social construction of parenthood" (ibid.).

This line of analysis underscores the need for a care*fair* policy strategy to engage in a contest of cultural politics to reconstruct the symbolic meaning of fatherhood. It is for this reason that I recommend linking participation in maternity and parental leave programs with eligibility for a public pension. In the Canadian context, every month of maternity or parental leave that someone takes should reduce by four months the total amount of (self-)employment that one must perform to qualify without penalty for benefits under the Canada or Quebec Pension Plan (C/QPP). If such a system were implemented, a parent who takes six months of leave following the birth of a child would qualify without penalty for C/QPP two years earlier than he or she would in the absence of taking this leave – at age sixty-three rather than sixty-five.

Under the current system, a citizen's CPP is reduced by 0.5 percent for every month she or he draws on the benefit program before turning sixty-five. Conversely, one's CPP increases by 0.5 percent for every month after sixty-five one delays receipt of benefits (up to a monthly maximum of $788.75). Thus, to claim the public pension at age sixty-three results in a 12 percent benefit penalty. Under care*fair*, if the same citizen took six months of maternity or parental leave, the reform I propose would eliminate this benefit reduction, since the point at which the person becomes eligible for a penalty-free CPP would drop by twenty-four months.

Pensions represent the social citizenship benefit that is most definitively linked to extensive work performance. Receiving a pension is a unique point in the adult life course when non-work becomes socially sanctioned in recognition of a successful history of productive contribution. ("For all you do, this pension's for you!" would be an appropriate slogan for CPP). By linking public pension entitlement to participation in maternity and parental leave programs, the care*fair* concept would make explicit that informal care provision is just as much a social responsibility as paid work. It would overtly signal that caregiving counts as critical work performance alongside labour force participation when the public determines eligibility for its paramount social citizenship benefit. A connection between parental leave and pensions would, thus, advance at the level of symbolic politics the idea that caregiving should count for masculine (not just feminine) ideals of work performance. At the very least, caregiving would become a contribution that the state would privilege relative to employment at a rate of one to four while the citizen is on a care leave, with the implication that employers should endeavour to accommodate more male participation in this mode of social (re)production.

The suggestion that one month of leave should count as four months of employment for public pension entitlement purposes is meant to serve as another plank on the path to restructuring the context of incentives in which citizens decide about time allocation for domestic care and labour force participation – a plank that would leave no doubt as to the state's intended symbolic message. The one-to-four ratio would also help to offset the dynamic consequences that result from labour market withdrawal for care purposes, including the pension penalty that primary caregivers have historically encountered as a result of weaker labour force attachment. As of October 2004, the average income that Canadian women earn from CPP retirement benefits is still under 60 percent of men's benefits: just $335 per month compared to $578 (Government of Canada 2004, Table 10). This pension disparity persists despite the fact that pension eligibility calculations exclude periods when mothers' earnings decline due to childrearing responsibilities for children under age seven. The care*fair* proposal to link caregiving leave to CPP calculations would partially address this disparity. Since a caregiver who takes six months of leave would reduce by twenty-four months the point at which she becomes eligible for C/QPP without penalty, a mother who works until age sixty-five would enjoy a 12 percent increase in her public pension compared to the status quo.

Care*fair* Reform 2: Paid Worktime Reductions over the Week and Year
In addition to reforming life-course employment norms to accommodate the social citizen who integrates caring and earning, a care*fair* policy framework would also revise employment norms over the week and year. This change would adapt policy models implemented in Germany and, especially, France. Both countries have instituted initiatives to reduce standard full-time work hours measured over a seven-day or annual period.

The French government introduced the *loi Aubry* in 1998. It launched a process that will see statutory weekly working time reduced from thirty-nine to thirty-five hours. The new legislation obliges employers to pay overtime premiums for weekly work following the thirty-sixth hour at a rate of 25 percent for the first seven hours and 50 percent for overtime hours thereafter. The premium can be taken as either added pay or time off, with a presumption in favour of time off in the absence of a collective agreement (Bilous 2000). The new French legislation also limits maximum annual overtime hours for individuals to 130 hours. This provision applies to professional staff and production managers but excludes senior management. Some intermediate-level managers have added flexibility under the statute, which permits up to 180 overtime hours per year (European Industrial Relations Review 2001c, 26-27).

The *loi Aubry* institutionalizes an annualized norm of working time that provides employers with new forms of flexibility in labour usage to facilitate compliance with the thirty-five-hour week (European Industrial Relations Review 1998, 22). Under this annual norm, the threshold after which overtime is calculated is 1,600 hours (European Industrial Relations Review 2001c, 27). The annualized norm permits employers to vary weekly working time according to demand and production cycles and facilitates the reduction of weekly working hours in the form of rest days. Rest days are specifically aimed to mitigate the problem of reducing the working time of executives, managers, and other senior staff by enabling companies to offer them time off in lieu of extra hours worked over given weeks. French legislation also allows rest days to be used in combination with a time-banking system that permits a share of time to be set aside for use over several years (European Industrial Relations Review 1998, 22).

While France pursued paid worktime reduction through legislation, Germany reduced full-time work norms through collective bargaining. Unions in Germany bargain at the industry level, and the terms of the collective contract apply not only to members but also to almost all other workers in the sector (Contensou and Vranceanu 2000, 36). In 1990 the union IG Metall and employers negotiated new initiatives to reduce hours of work to thirty-five per week (from 38.5) without loss of pay but with a slower pace of wage increase. In return, employers received more flexibility in the organization of the manufacturing process, which permits capital to be used for longer hours and on weekends in order to avoid overtime payments (J. Hunt 1998). By early 1995, ten industrial sectors in Germany covering 6.5 million workers signed similar worktime frameworks (Contensou and Vranceanu 2000, 37).

A care*fair* regime that adapts the French and German models would explicitly reverse many of the recent employment standard revisions in Ontario and British Columbia that enable companies to rely on individual employees for longer hours. The policy would apply overtime premiums starting in the thirty-sixth hour of work per week (averaged over a year), in contrast to current provincial arrangements that stipulate overtime premiums will be paid after between forty and forty-eight hours (Hayden 1999, 116). The shift to shorter work hours could retain the time-and-a-half regular pay overtime premium typical in most provinces or implement a tiered overtime system as in France.

A reduction in statutory full-time hours would track the Canadian labour market shift across occupational categories in the 1990s that saw proportionately more citizens find positions with workweeks shorter, rather than longer, than thirty-five hours (Hall 1999, 33). Since shorter employment hours in Canada presently imply significant social costs for some workers in the form of few, if any, fringe benefits and social protections, policies designed to normalize reduced full-time hours should be accompanied by measures that mitigate this trend. In 2002 the Government of Saskatchewan (2002) implemented legislation that provides a useful model to explore further. Labour standards in that province now entitle employees who work at least thirty hours a week in businesses with ten or more full-time equivalents to participate fully in the dental, prescription, and insurance benefit programs offered to colleagues working longer hours. The legislation also entitles part-time workers who labour fifteen to thirty hours a week to 50 percent of a company's benefit program.

The general reduction of full-time paid work hours over the week or year institutionalized in France and Germany constitutes an important strategy for remedying the functional division between breadwinner and unpaid caregiver, even though the policies do not specifically target the needs of parents of young children. Household decisions regarding the division of care are dynamic rather than static choices. The term "dynamic" acknowledges that such decisions have considerable influence on future work options, wages, and pension entitlements, just as choices regarding levels of education, skills development, and length of tenure at a particular workplace do. Persons fulfilling the primary care role risk enduring harmful economic consequences that manifest themselves in, among other things, occupational segregation and shorter hours of paid work that account for 10 and 15 percent of the gender earnings gap in Canada respectively (Cleveland and Krashinsky 1998, 43). The earnings gap, in turn, contributes to less valuable pensions and higher rates of poverty among senior women as compared to senior men. Thus, while about one in five families in Canada has a child under six at any given time, the dynamic nature of decisions about the division of care means that employment norms regulating hours of work have long-term consequences for the roughly 80 percent of Canadians who have children at some point in their lives.

Caregiving is also not just about preschool-age children. Citizens are always persons in relations, and careloads wax and wane during different life-course stages. Census data from 2001 showed that 46 percent of labour force participants have children residing at home, and 19 percent provide some elder care.[3] The previous census revealed that 20 percent of labour force participants shoulder both roles.[4] While this book has focused predominantly on child care issues, social care responsibilities exist in regard to adult dependants as well. The inverted population pyramid will only increase elder care responsibilities and the particular challenges encountered by the sandwich generation as baby boomers continue to retire over the next decades, and younger employees delay having children (Duxbury and Higgins 2003, 14). Thus, in addition to the dynamic consequences of decisions about childrearing arrangements, caregiving aspirations and obligations are lifelong issues that mitigate participation across social spaces.

Revising employment standards also has the potential to reorganize the financial incentives to which citizens respond. Shorter standard hours imply, on average, a more significant decline in income for men compared to women. In Canada, men work overtime more regularly than women, accounting for almost two in three overtime hours (Duchesne 1997, 10-11). Similarly, fathers of preschoolers in dual-earner heterosexual couples in which both parents are employed full-time work for pay 10.5 more hours a week than mothers (Silver 2000, 27). A reduction in standard working hours will, therefore, have a particularly significant effect on men's paid work patterns, decreasing their average hours and earnings proportionately more than women's. As a result, paid-working-time transitions would shift the balance of existing economic incentives within heterosexual couples. Reduced earnings for men may generate an income effect, in response to which women who currently do not perform full-time paid work hours may increase the time they dedicate to employment. The extent of the income effect will be mediated by the degree to which spouses are substitutes in caregiving and household production. It will also be affected by the importance of complementarity in leisure that may incline some spouses to respond to a partner's added leisure by retaining or reducing their own level of paid work so that the couple can enjoy unpaid time together (J. Hunt 1998).

The proposal to reduce full-time employment norms will by no means preclude part-time hours. Shorter or casual work arrangements are attractive to firms pressured to compete by employing a just-in-time workforce that can be manipulated in cost-effective ways to respond to the ups and downs of the production and product delivery cycles, as well as to consumer demands. The firms' search for labour flexibility will, therefore, be a primary factor driving persistent growth in part-time hours. However, shorter hours will also continue to hold out for some women (and men) an opportunity to reconcile competing care-giving and career goals, particularly in the current context, where quality, affordable child care programs are in short supply in Canada and other liberal welfare regimes. The goal to ensure citizens have adequate time to interweave domestic activities with other citizenry pursuits would thus be advanced by following Sweden, which has institutionalized a right to shorter workweeks for parents of young children (O'Hara 1998, 16). Legislation that grants parents a right to shorter work schedules of thirty hours (or four days) a week until children reach age seven would cater more to individual choices regarding work-life balance. If something like the Saskatchewan government's policy regulating employment benefits were implemented across the country, thirty-hour weekly employment schedules (averaged over a year) would still entitle the citizen to the full range of benefits offered to full-time employees.

So long as part-time work remains prominent, there will be a risk of gender inequality premised on the functional division between primary earner and primary caregiver. The risks are minimized, however, the more that the functional division between earning and caring is bridged. The bridge is made increasingly secure as persons with considerable unpaid care work, including lone mothers, are better positioned to serve as core employees, who closely approximate the hours on the job typical of childless staff or of staff who do not share primary responsibility for their children. A reduction in standard full-time hours to 1,600 per year raises the probability that this challenging balancing act will become a genuine opportunity for citizens.

Care*fair* Reform 3: Enriched Public Commitments to Child Care
A third policy trajectory required by a care*fair* framework would render paid labour market participation more compatible with unpaid caregiving ambitions and responsibilities by implementing far stronger public commitments to child care services. Federal, provincial, and territorial governments in Canada should collaborate to inject substantially more public funding into regulated child care services so that the state subsidizes roughly 80 percent of the costs of care for all children under six. This level of state funding would be consistent with expenditures in Denmark and France, and is also being institutionalized in the province of Quebec.

The Quebec child care system has two parts that are relevant to children under six (Tougas 2002, Chapter 1). The first provides full-school-day kindergarten programs for all five-year-olds, with no parent fees. The second subsidizes child care organized by Centres de la petite enfance (CPEs), which coordinate full-day programs in centres for children from birth to age four, as well as programs in home-based family day care contexts for children under thirteen. The maximum cost of full-day care in both settings is $7 per day, regardless of a family's income or employment status. The $7 daily parent fee covers roughly 20 percent of the actual cost of care, with the provincial government paying the remaining operating expenses.

While other provinces may prefer a different fee system than that implemented in Quebec, all should adopt some version of a sliding fee scale to ensure that no family would be responsible for more than 30 percent of actual costs, following the Danish model (Esping-Andersen 2002, 61; Moss and Penn 1996, 123). Before establishing new government funding levels, average caregiver wages in provinces other than Quebec should be reviewed and increased (in Quebec they were raised by roughly 40 percent in 1999) to ensure that child care workers do not subsidize care arrangements for parents and the state through low wages. Pay inequity is a pervasive problem in the child care sector. Cleveland and Hyatt (2002, 577-78) find that, "on average, female workers with similar education get paid nearly 40 per cent more annually than female child care workers for full-time work."

Extending Quebec's child care model across Canada would represent a dramatic departure from the existing funding scheme in many provinces. As of 1998, parent fees cover, on average, 82 percent of actual regulated care costs in Newfoundland; more than two-thirds of costs in the Maritimes; half of costs in British Columbia, Alberta, and Ontario; and 38 and 34 percent in Saskatchewan and Manitoba respectively (Childcare Resource and Research Unit 2000, 108).

The commitment to subsidize spaces for all children under six would require an even more dramatic increase in the number of regulated spaces. There are regulated spaces in Canada for just 12 percent of all children under age twelve as of 2001. Outside Quebec, the rate ranges from as low as 4 percent in Saskatchewan to 14 percent in PEI (Friendly, Beach, and Turiano 2002, 156). Quebec stands out for having spaces for 21 percent of children. Nevertheless, the still-inadequate supply of spaces is a significant problem with the $7-per-day Quebec child care system, as Baril, Lefebvre, and Merrigan (2000) have charged. The provincial government had a plan to partially address this problem by creating an additional 67,000 regulated spaces between 2001 and 2006 – a goal that was well within reach, given that annual growth in regulated spaces since the universal program was launched surpassed 16 percent (Government of Quebec 2001, 17). However, the status of this plan is uncertain as a result of the election of the Charest Liberal government in 2003.

The net cost of a pan-Canadian child care system that subsidizes fees by approximately 80 percent would be substantial. Cleveland and Krashinsky (1998) estimate the cost of a system available to children between the ages of two and five inclusive as $7.91 billion annually (less than 0.8 percent of GDP), approximately $5.3 billion a year more than federal and provincial governments spent on child care as of 1997. The Cleveland and Krashinsky study concludes that the additional $5.3 billion will eventually generate more than $10.5 billion in annual benefits in terms of better early childhood development outcomes and increased female labour force participation – a favourable two-to-one benefit/cost ratio. The initial injection of $5.3 billion in new public expenditures implies higher marginal tax rates (MTRs) over a transition period before the anticipated positive consequences of increased child care spending materialize. The Cleveland and Krashinsky analysis does not attempt to estimate adverse effects on economic efficiency associated with higher MTRs during this interim period. However, the projected two-to-one benefit/cost ratio suggests that increased investment in quality child care has the potential to lower MTRs over the medium and long terms, generating efficiency gains beyond those projected by Cleveland and Krashinsky.

Although child care policy will not directly provide people with more affordable time outside of the labour market, it is nonetheless an integral piece of a care*fair* policy platform because of its potential to challenge the gender division of care within heterosexual couples. Research regularly identifies a strong connection between women's labour force attachment and the share of care and domestic work that male spouses shoulder (for example, Coltrane 1996; Sanderson and Thompson 2002). Generally, the more women contribute to overall household income, the greater share of domestic work their husbands perform. Men's share of housework and caregiving also tends to rise as women demonstrate a longer period of continuous paid workforce experience and as their occupational prestige increases relative to that of their husbands. The correlation between women's labour force attachment and men's contributions to the domestic sphere suggest that women are better positioned to demand that spouses share care and domestic duties as the women's relative earnings potential rises. A higher female earnings potential also means that heterosexual couples have less reason to limit specifically the market participation of wives for the purpose of supporting the employment success of husbands or for saving child care and other domestic expenses. The additional earnings that typically accompany women's stronger attachment to the paid labour force may also provide male partners with added financial security, which in turn could permit men to reduce their paid worktime and shoulder a greater share of the domestic workload.

This research supports significantly increasing funding for child care arrangements if minimizing gender inequality is a public policy priority. Econometric findings by Cleveland, Gunderson, and Hyatt (1996) and Powell (1997), which were discussed above, reveal the negative influence that child care costs exert on the labour supply of mothers. In light of their calculations and the average cost of full-day regulated care in British Columbia, the introduction of a $7-per-day child care system can be expected to increase the probability that BC mothers will accept paid work by between 27 and 30 percent. Some US econometric literature suggests that the positive employment influence of lower child care fees will be even greater among single and low-income mothers (for a review, see Baum 2002, 140-41).

The correlation between female labour force attachment and male assumption of domestic duties also provides strong reason to limit new funding for child care exclusively to regulated arrangements, despite charges that such a policy is not neutral with respect to parental preferences about earning and caring. Baril, Lefebvre, and Merrigan (2000, 10) raise this concern in regard to the Quebec child care system. They argue that it is "for the most part benefiting families where the parents [are] participating in the labour market." A more neutral system, they maintain, would not unduly influence parental choices by "passing any value judgement as to families' lifestyle preferences" (26).

In place of Quebec's child care arrangement, Baril, Lefebvre, and Merrigan (2000, 26) recommend that the same funding be used to introduce "a nontaxable universal family allowance." They offer two options: the first, a demogrant of $1,752 annually per child under eighteen; the second, a tiered universal allowance system of $2,754 for children under six, and $1,377 for children ages seven to fifteen. Both proposals would provide more cash in hand for parents with children, increasing the resources and giving them the choice to remain home with their children or go to work and hire child care services.

The Baril, Lefebvre, and Merrigan critique is seriously flawed, however. It wrongly presupposes that the social, economic, and policy contexts prior to the introduction of the new child care program in Quebec were neutral with regard to families' caregiving decisions. This assumption ignores the historical evolution of social institutions in response to the patriarchal division of labour. The early postwar era assigned primary responsibility for caregiving, both ideologically and practically, to diverse groups of women, withdrawing funding for child care following the Second World War (Baker 1995, 199) and recruiting female foreign domestics (Arat-Koc 1997). Labour market expectations about ideal workers were constructed by men, based on male experience, and produced employment norms regarding hours of work that are largely incompatible with primary responsibility for unpaid caring (Slaughter 1995). Early postwar attitudes depicted women in the labour market as secondary earners and less productive due to pregnancy and their primary childrearing roles (Pateman 1989, 190). Girls were (and still are) socialized to assume domestic roles as wives and mothers and thus were often encouraged to invest less in human capital, while social expectations about appropriate occupations for women contributed to employment segregation (Phillips and Phillips 1993, 60). Each of these factors contributed to a gender earnings differential that powers a self-reinforcing cycle in which, as we have seen, it becomes economically "rational" for heterosexual couples to maximize household income by investing more heavily in the man's career and the woman's domesticity.

The proposal to replace Quebec's child care system with a demogrant that is ostensibly more neutral ignores the systemic forces that underpin this cycle and, as a result, fails to challenge them.[5] Added cash in hand for both familial and non-familial care does not provide incentives that encourage women's labour force ties or men's attachment to unpaid care responsibilities. Since families will receive the subsidy regardless of labour force patterns, women's after-tax earnings must still surpass the cost of care arrangements and lost domestic productivity before some couples will think it financially worthwhile for mothers to pursue paid employment. The maximum $2,754 value of the proposed allowance also falls well short of the average annual cost of regulated care ($5,928 to $8,460 for full day care in British Columbia), increasing the risk that couples will decide that it is not worth having two earners, given child care costs, employment expenses, taxes, lost domestic productivity, and lost household time. As a result, the Baril, Lefebvre, and Merrigan proposal is more likely to shift the balance of incentives further toward supporting one parent (typically the mother) in dual-parent families to withdraw from the labour force by adding an additional few thousand dollars to ease this transition. With such decisions, the patriarchal division of care labour is buttressed rather than challenged. By contrast, the Quebec child care system institutionalizes new incentives that mitigate systemic factors underpinning patriarchy because they explicitly reduce the relative cost of non-familial care, thereby encouraging stronger labour market ties for women.

Duty Discourse and Choice

Care*fair* is by no means neutral about the choices men should make. The resulting policy changes would acknowledge that caregiving is a social responsibility equal to employment and payment of taxes. The objective is to encourage men to rescind the patriarchal dividend by performing an equitable share of care.

This departure from neutrality is a response to recent work by Olson (2002). He develops a cogent analysis of the difficulties that confront any social movement committed to challenging the gender division of care. Advocates of a universal caregiver model, he observes, confront a circular relation between the choices that individuals make and prescriptive cultural norms. Before men will choose, en masse, to care more, cultural norms about masculinity, fatherhood, motherhood, and employment must evolve to endorse male caregiving as a valuable practice on a par with other citizenry pursuits that enjoy more social status for men. Before such norms become solidly woven into the cultural fabric, however, men must start to care more. The circular relation thus gives rise to the problem of the chicken or the egg: which change will occur first?

The care*fair* framework I outline in this chapter aims to address the circular relation by employing public policy levers to nudge men to make more socially responsible and equitable choices about caregiving. The nudge remains a relatively gentle one, since under care*fair*, men would not be forced to care more. They may still choose to continue current care patterns, but there would be new consequences, such as postponed eligibility for a full public pension and the loss of leave benefits. Thus, care*fair* would not so much compel care activity as it would change the system of incentives within which men make choices between market and domestic activities.

This level of persuasion stands in contrast to the level of coercion that Mead (1997b) advocates in his paternalist vision of workfare. In his preferred category of paternalist policies that enforce compliance, he does not include reforms that redesign policy incentives to encourage work. He believes that tinkering with policy incentives still "leave[s] work as a choice" (47). Since Mead rejects the competence assumption, he is not confident that individuals will respond to policy-induced economic incentives, even when incentives make paid work in their self-interest. He therefore concludes that an effective workfare scheme must go beyond reordering policy incentives to coerce citizens to work more directly through supervision.

The care*fair* reforms I have proposed in this chapter do not entail the level of supervised coercion that Mead urges. Nonetheless, they remain out of step with the work of Olson (2002, 387), who is skeptical about employing even the modest level of policy influence that care*fair* prescribes. "*Choice* is a key element of ... [a democratic political] system," he maintains. "Democrats see the state as a choice-promoting institution, one that opens up a wide variety of life options for its citizens rather than dictating particular forms of life to them. Any such state would have to countenance a certain amount of choice in the benefits people receive. For instance, universal caregiver would presumably permit people to choose their own mix of care-giving labor, other forms of labor and leisure. Presumably it would allow people to choose whether their caregiving takes the form of official economic work or informal work."

Olson adds that we should be cautious about the kinds of care*fair* reforms I propose because they may constrain individual choice. He rejects the proposal to reserve some months of parental leave exclusively for fathers on the grounds that it "introduces a substantial amount of paternalism into welfare, stipulating social relations in a way that welfare theorists find quite problematic in other contexts" (2002, 394). Similarly, he argues that the recommendation to shorten the workweek so that overtime costs arise after fewer hours of employment would be problematic "because it would discriminate against wage earners relative to salary earners. A man on an annual salary could easily avoid the state's system of costs and incentives simply because his work hours are contractually open-ended and his salary is fixed" (ibid.). In Olson's view, both policy proposals are inadequate because they are "circumscribed by their economic character and by their entanglement in issues of class. They pursue gender equity by modifying the structural circumstances in which people act. They do not, however, directly modify the social and cultural bases of choice in the use of social services" (395).

The charge that revised employment standards will disproportionately affect the choices of waged workers over salaried employees has merit. It is not obvious, however, that policy makers should resist the larger care*fair* strategy to transform the patriarchal division of care just because a single aspect of the reform agenda is likely to target one class of men over another. Olson's class-based analysis is also misguided when it addresses parental leave. In contrast to his supposition that the policy will target working-class waged employees more directly, studies of parental leave in Scandinavian countries show that the daddy month experiment has disproportionately encouraged higher-income fathers to care more, especially those who work in the public sector (for example, Leira 1998, 370).

Despite the limitations of Olson's class analysis, his attention to the diversity of male experience, including class differences, is important, as both Connell (1995) and Coltrane (1996) have argued. The more problematic element of Olson's article is, instead, that his preferred policy reforms to remedy the patriarchal dividend are weak and undeveloped at best, and inconsistent with his analysis at worst. In place of redesigning employment standards and leave benefits, Olson would abandon the project of reorganizing financial incentives in favour of two strategies that concentrate on cultural politics to restructure gender norms. The first is education policy (2002, 401-2). He would manipulate school curriculum to articulate gender equality norms that challenge the legacy of patriarchy. The second strategy would increase women's relative bargaining position within the family by promoting their labour market options and "forcing men to bear a greater part of domestic burdens" to decrease "the subsidized labor market mobility they have long enjoyed" (402).

The latter suggestion is somewhat perplexing in light of Olson's emphasis on choice: the language of "force" is clearly inconsistent with this. What is more, how does he propose to compel men to bear a greater share of domestic burdens if not by restructuring economic incentives through changes to policy that regulates full-time norms and parental leave? Olson is, unfortunately, silent about this issue, other than suggesting that men must be socialized to become caregivers through (moral) education. There is no doubt that education will play a significant role in the transformation and redefinition of gender norms. Research indicates that men's education is a strong predictor of men's use of parental leave (Bergman and Hobson 2002, 117; Leira 1998, 370), as well as a predictor of the propensity for men to share domestic care work more generally (Walker and McGraw 2000, 567). Nevertheless, the singular reliance that Olson places on education to recalibrate the gender order bears strong resemblance to the trepidation that Kymlicka and Norman report about authors addressing citizenship issues when it comes to applying their theories to public policy. Olson offers an insightful analysis but draws the wrong policy conclusions. There is no place for timidity in a universal caregiver framework.

Olson's focus on choice is a helpful reminder, however, of the fact that policy prescriptions suitable for social democratic and corporatist regimes in Europe are not obviously culturally appropriate in their liberal welfare regime cousins. Esping-Andersen's (1990, 1999) formative regime-cluster work provides strong support for the claim that Canada, the United States, Australia, New Zealand, and Great Britain diverge importantly from their continental European counterparts in terms of the primacy they assign to the marketplace to mediate the distribution of welfare across society. On one hand, a preoccupation with market efficiency motivates a stronger cultural commitment in Anglo-speaking nations to a circumscribed state that primarily regulates the relations of exchange and enforces property rights in social conditions of scarcity. The shift to weaker employment standards regulating maximum hours of paid work in Ontario and British Columbia is an example of this trend. On the other hand, the preoccupation with market forces underpins a more cautious approach to social benefits on the grounds that they may generate incentives that incline citizens to opt for state assistance over waged work. The resulting preference for a smaller state role in social service delivery explains, in part, the tepid public funding of parental leave and child care programs provided in Canada compared to many European countries.

The liberal welfare culture is a reality of the Canadian policy arena. Policy innovation stands a greater chance of succeeding, therefore, if it works to embrace one or more key norms that inform the cultural context. Recall the insight about counterhegemony that Gramsci's (1971) theorizing motivates: a paradigm is only hegemonic because it resonates (at least in part) with much of the citizenry, including those who are ultimately disadvantaged by the paradigm. Thus, the path to replacing a hegemonic paradigm does not lie so much in negating it as in refashioning critical elements in order to reprioritize values that are currently missing and to relocate or exhaust problematic features that are prominent.

Here lies the unique opportunity that the shift toward duty discourses presents for proponents of care*fair*. In contrast to Olson's (2002, 394) claim that the use of state power to privilege some social choices over others introduces a level of paternalism into public policy that welfare theorists "find quite problematic in other contexts," citizens of liberal regimes (re-)elect policy makers who employ the authoritative power of the state to compel citizens to discharge social duties in respect of paid work. Using the same state authority to enforce citizenry care obligations can therefore be presented as a logical next step in this cultural milieu. Although the punitive character of some workfare policies appropriately draws criticism (for example, Klein and Long 2003), it turns out that the neoliberal concern with moral hazard and public enforcement of social obligations offers an especially solid cornerstone for developing, in liberal regimes, a gender-equality framework premised on the universal caregiver model.

Assigning to the state an important role in obliging citizens invokes a now well-accepted Weberian analysis of the state, as Taylor-Goodby (1991, 208) has noted. He observes that "many definitions of the state do not pay much attention to the meeting of citizens' needs, but all put the 'monopoly on the legitimate use of violence within a given territory,' in Weber's terminology, at their heart. Welfare states are not simply about doing good to individuals by meeting their needs, they are about sanctioning, controlling and directing people's behaviour as well."

Sanctions and controls are vital to the state, even in the liberal tradition, because the state functions as protector and guarantor of individual liberty. A government must rightfully exercise its power to limit a citizen's activity against his or her will whenever that activity encroaches on the liberty of others or otherwise inflicts injury. This insight is the foundation of John Stuart Mill's (1975, 10-11) famous harm principle, which argues that "the only purpose for which power can be rightfully exercised over any member of a civilized community, against his will, is to prevent harm to others."

The harm principle, in turn, illuminates the linchpin for defending the position that welfare state policy is an appropriate mechanism for addressing the gender division of labour. The perverse incentives that perpetuate male free riding on the care work of diverse groups of women undermine equality of opportunity and place women at risk of economic insecurity and marginalization from important social areas. The solution to this moral hazard demands a vision of social citizenship entitlements that institutionalizes sanctions as much as benefits, just as the harm principle prescribes use of state authority to shield individual liberty. Borrowing from Taylor-Goodby (1991, 208), we must recognize that "equal enjoyment of rights requires that some people should be prevented from infringing the human need for freedom of others by not participating in the paid and unpaid work that is necessary to the continuance of society."

The institutional redesign proposed by the care*fair* framework is also consistent with the sort of restructuring that T.H. Marshall (1964) and John Rawls (1971) imply is necessary to facilitate genuine social inclusion. Recall that both maintain that dignified social membership demands that major institutions comply with the standard of civilization Marshall advances or the difference principle Rawls defends. Since society represents a system of cooperation without which no single individual alone could lead a satisfactory life, both theorists call for institutions to be reorganized so that they draw forth (even if only hypothetically) the voluntary cooperation of all citizens, including the less advantaged. It is not reasonable to presume, however, that all individuals would voluntarily participate in society if the social order is premised on the idea that certain social locations exist to serve others at the expense of the person providing the service. Yet this is precisely what a gender division of care allows. Similarly, with the difference principle and the standard of civilization, Rawls and Marshall speak out against a social order that permits some individuals to suffer a relative level of inequality in income, wealth, and/or power that impedes their substantive equality of opportunity. Again, this consequence is exactly the penalty that women suffer in a world where men's irresponsibility for care represents a patriarchal dividend. Redesigning state institutions to entice, or even compel, men to rescind their privilege of irresponsibility is therefore an implication that follows from the analytic thrust evident in Marshall's and Rawls's foundational work on social citizenship, regardless of the limitations that their own patriarchal assumptions imposed on their analyses.

The imperative to oblige men to care more is also implicit, but undeveloped, in S. White's (2000, 2003) discussion of the intuitive conditions for fair reciprocity that a just system of welfare contractualism requires. While neoliberalism presumes that anyone who willingly shares in the mutual advantages made possible by society's cooperative venture has an obligation to make a reasonable productive contribution to the community in return, White's (2000, 515-16, 134-35) research suggests that this reciprocity principle cannot legitimately bind citizens irrespective of the society's institutional structures. A number of social conditions must first exist. He identifies the following conditions: a minimum standard of productive participation should guarantee all citizens a decent share of the social product; all citizens should enjoy decent opportunities to engage in productive participation; all citizens (capable of production) should be forced to comply with the minimum standard of productive participation; and different forms of productive participation should be treated equally (ibid.).

When caregiving is evaluated in light of these conditions, it is apparent that domestic care labour is not treated on a par with paid employment in modern capitalist societies. Many men are not culturally expected to make a productive contribution to the social product by fulfilling a reasonable share of care duties. The gender division of care makes it more challenging for women to attain a decent share of the social product through employment, at the same time that social institutions in liberal welfare regimes deliver only minimal remuneration to persons who specialize in domestic caregiving. Inequalities in income further obstruct some citizens from enjoying sufficient opportunities to contribute to domestic care because financial need imposes time constraints, while employment norms prescribe very long hours for the most valued labour market participants.

The attention to securing decent opportunities for all citizens to make a productive contribution, including through caregiving, once again reminds us that care*fair* is not just about preventing harm. It also takes seriously that there is inequality in opportunity to care, one that some poor women and women of colour suffer, as discussed in Chapter 6. Many men also endure this inequality as a consequence of their patriarchal privileges. Limited domestic participation may mean that some men do not cultivate care ambitions and thus risk compromising their social memberships. Research by Eggebeen and Knoester (2001) confirms this exclusion. Their quantitative analysis found that, among men living with their biological or adopted children, fathers' "level of involvement with their children made a substantial difference" to activities well beyond child rearing (389). "The more these men were engaged in activities with their children, the more satisfied they were with their lives, the more socializing they did, the more involved they were in their communities, [and] the more connected they were to their families" (ibid.).

Thus, the authoritative "stick" that care*fair* brings to public policy has the potential to produce positive spinoff consequences for social inclusion among many of the men whose behaviour it aims to alter most. There are other benefits, in addition to challenging male exclusion, that can be expected from care*fair* reforms, which are explored in more detail in the next chapter. I give particular attention to benefits that arise in respect of socioeconomic problems that are more likely to motivate policy innovation in the present political milieu than is the objective of gender equality.

8
The Politics of Time[1]

The pervasiveness of duty discourse across disparate schools of political thought offers one strategic opening for advocates of gender equality to sell the merits of a care*fair* reform agenda. The reorganization of public policy to oblige citizens to discharge social duties is incomplete so long as care responsibilities are ignored. The same logic of reciprocity that underpins workfare also behooves us to address men's privilege of irresponsibility for care.

Still, we should not be sanguine about the modest attention that gender equality attracts among architects of welfare state redesign in Canada and other liberal welfare regimes. The work of Courchene (1994a, 2001) and Richards (1997) is instructive on this point. Richards, we have seen, discounts the search for gender equality as a "special interest" and questions how inegalitarian the postwar family ideal of a primary breadwinner/primary caregiver was for women (54, 211). Courchene (esp. 1994a), by contrast, subscribes to an individual responsibility model of the family that largely ignores the many barriers impeding extensive paid work for primary carers, as well as the costs that many women endure as a result of the gender division of care. In both cases the result is that Courchene and Richards recommend policy blueprints to guide recalibration of Canadian social policy that are silent about labour standards regulating full-time norms and engage only minimally with questions of employment leave or child care. Gender equality simply does not register as a priority on their policy radar.

This silence renders Courchene's and Richards's reform proposals inadequate in terms of gender equality. While this shortcoming is a problem for social justice, it also restricts their ability to address social and economic problems that extend well beyond the analytic boundaries typically assigned to questions of women's equality. In this chapter, I defend care*fair* as a key building block for social citizenship infrastructure on the grounds that dismantling the legacy of patriarchy has potential to address, at least partially, a wide range of socioeconomic challenges. Problems include the decline in real wages for men, the associated shift in poverty to families with young children, the resulting adverse consequences for future human capital, anticipated labour shortages, earnings polarization, and persistent un(der)employment.

Proponents of the third way are increasingly sensitive to this potential. The child-centred social investment strategy and new gender contract that Esping-Andersen (2002) advocates identify child care as a key foundation for a recast welfare system. This is an especially strong element of his analysis, to which I return below to offer additional support. But the strength of Esping-Andersen's child care analysis also reflects the one-sided workerist vision of social inclusion with which he operates. Child care is emphasized to promote inclusion in the marketplace for mothers today and for children tomorrow. Policies that promote time outside the market are left unexplored in Esping-Andersen's third way analysis, despite the fact that he acknowledges the growing polarization between work-poor and work-rich households (39-50). This chapter aims to remedy Esping-Andersen's oversight by placing far more emphasis than he does on work-life balance through employment leave policies and labour standards that would shorten full-time work norms. While these policy alternatives do not represent a panacea for all that ails postindustrial societies, they offer opportunities to address some of the deleterious socioeconomic consequences that are associated with polarization in the distribution of paid worktime.

This deviation from the third way urges renewed interest in what I refer to as the politics of time. The term "politics" acknowledges that public policy mediates citizens' access to paid and unpaid temporal opportunities. The level of demand for employment, and its distribution between citizens, are significantly influenced by state regulations governing employment standards and industrial relations, monetary and taxation policies, and social spending. Non-labour-market time is also affected by state decommodification measures that moderate the degree to which citizens can maintain their livelihood without selling their labour.

The public role in fostering employment, regulating labour market practices, and decommodifying citizens renders time, whether it is paid time in the market or unpaid time across other key social spaces, a divisible social benefit. Individual patterns of time usage are not simply a matter of personal prerogative, but also a function of social decisions. As such, questions of distributive justice arise regarding citizens' access

to diverse time-related opportunities, including the potential harmful-
ness of time constraints and imbalances that impede individual participation in important areas of community life. Given the significance of
time in the labour market and the domestic sphere for full community
membership, the collective interest in distributive justice should extend
beyond the allocation of material rewards to account also for the distribution of time for paid work, family, and other citizenship practices.

Human-Capital Development
The child-centred welfare strategy that Esping-Andersen (2002) defends
invokes a life-course perspective to illuminate "the real importance of
investing in the well-being and resources of children" (27). This perspective is informed by a burgeoning neuroscience literature, which reveals "that the early years of development from conception to age six,
particularly for the first three years, set the base for competence and
coping skills that will affect learning, behaviour and health throughout
life" (Norrie McCain and Mustard 1999, 5). One implication is that social exclusion emerges as a problem for many citizens by the time they
reach kindergarten, since some children are more ready for school than
others. Research by Hertzman (2002) shows that readiness to learn and
engage socially is not randomly distributed across Canadian society; it
follows a systematic pattern that is predictable. When we examine socioeconomic data, moving from children of the wealthiest and most educated families, through those from the middle, and on to those from
families with the least income and education, it is apparent that an
increasing share of children from less-well-off households are vulnerable in terms of school readiness. Hertzman refers to this pattern, in
which "risk increases in a stepwise fashion as one descends the socioeconomic ladder," as a "gradient," and states that "the gradient in child
development is an important aspect of social exclusion because, once
established, it tracks across the life course. Those who enter school in a
vulnerable state will tend to be less healthy, experience lower levels of
well-being, and be more likely to end up in socially marginal positions
as life unfolds" (1).

   It is difficult to compensate later in the life course for the harm done
in childhood. Remedial policies that target socially excluded youth and
adults are less effective than policies designed to foster early childhood
welfare, and remedial policies are often more expensive (Heckman and
Lochner 2000). There are, thus, strong reasons to invest in the early
years of citizenry development if human-capital accumulation is a public
policy priority. As Esping-Andersen (2002, 55) comments, "if childhood

poverty translates into less education, inferior cognitive skills, more criminality, and inferior lives, the secondary effect is a mass of low-productivity workers, highly vulnerable to unemployment and low pay in the 'new economy.' They will yield less revenue to tax authorities and probably require more public aid during their active years." He argues that "a concerted child-focus is," therefore, "*sine qua non* for a sustainable, efficient, and competitive knowledge-based production system. The coming working-age cohorts will be small, and they must sustain huge retirement populations. The income security of pensioners two or three decades down the line will in large measure depend on how much we can mobilize the productive potential of those who today are children. More generally, the only real asset that most advanced nations hold is the quality and skills of their people" (28).

Since available evidence indicates that the early years are a critical juncture for human-capital development, our systems of social protection and investment must evolve to address the shift in low-income status from the elderly toward young families with children. Cross-nationally, the Organisation for Economic Co-operation and Development (1999, 65) reports that "there is a generalised worsening of the position of those in households with a young head. Households with children are doing noticeably less well than previously in several countries. This contrasts with an improvement in the position of the elderly."

In Canada, the deteriorating fortunes of young families reflect in part the steady decline in real wages suffered by male labour market entrants since 1970. As discussed earlier, Beaudry and Green (2000) find that a university-educated male entrant in 1992 earned approximately 20 percent less than his counterpart did twenty years earlier. He also had little hope of enjoying eventual compensation for his lower initial wages through receipt of greater or more frequent wage increases in recognition of added experience over time.

In response, enriched child care and parental leave provisions have the potential to mediate some of the added challenges that younger workers encounter as a result of declining real starting wages and slower wage growth. Both policies can operate as keenly timed citizenship entitlements that preserve or supplement household income at periods when private expenses are particularly high and income is often relatively low. The care*fair* reforms to child care and parental leave proposed in the previous chapter would allow some of the extra costs associated with childrearing (whether forgone income due to labour market withdrawal or expenditures on services) to be spread over the life cycle and repaid through income taxes on a sliding scale sensitive to income as one's paid worklife proceeds.

Quality, affordable child care will be particularly important for defending against the deleterious developmental consequences of growing up amidst poverty. Indirectly, child care protects against the risks of stunted child development, to which poverty gives rise, by facilitating maternal employment. In light of declining real wages for men, maternal employment is now perhaps the most effective bulwark against child poverty. The National Council of Welfare (2002, Table 8.3) reports that the percentage of Canadian husband-wife households with children under six that fall below the poverty line before taxes would rise from 7 to 21 percent in the absence of maternal earnings (for a cross-national analysis of the same theme, see Esping-Andersen 2002, Table 2.8). The effectiveness of maternal employment as a strategy to reduce child poverty will only grow as non-parental care services become more affordable and mothers are financially able to sustain stronger attachment to the labour market.

The need for affordable child care to facilitate maternal employment is particularly evident with respect to lone mothers in Canada, more than half of whom fall below low-income cut-offs before taxes (National Council of Welfare 2002, Figure 3.1). Of these mothers, just 54 percent report any earnings, and the average value is less than $8,000 (Table 4.4). In contrast, in Sweden, where child care provisions are far more generous and accessible than in Canada, lone mothers have stronger labour market attachments and report market earnings as their main source of income more regularly. The result is that just one-third of single mothers in Sweden have pre-transfer incomes below the poverty line, and only 5 percent remain below this line after taxes and transfers (Sainsbury 1996, 84). In the absence of maternal employment, the story in Sweden would be very different. Esping-Andersen (2002, Table 2.4) calculates that the odds of lone-parent poverty in Sweden rise by over 117 percent if the mother does not work.

Beyond facilitating maternal employment, quality child care can also directly counter the ill consequences of low income by stimulating healthy development. Data from the Canadian National Longitudinal Survey of Children and Youth reveal that maternal participation in the labour market has a minimal effect on the school readiness scores of most preschool children (Gagné 2003), even though Canada does not have a child care system that reliably provides quality care. The one modest influence discovered is among children of parents with above-average parenting skills and levels of education – parents who, we can presume, are more likely to read to their children and provide social and educational stimuli. Such children "tend to benefit slightly more in terms of cognitive skills from additional parental time than children of less skilled parents" (33).

This research points to the importance that quality care plays in child development, regardless of whether the setting is parental or non-parental. Just as children benefit from more time with skilled-parent caregivers, results from the US Cost, Quality and Child Outcomes (CQO) study (Peisner-Feinberg et al. 1999, 7-8) show that children who attend higher-quality centres benefit from better levels of school readiness upon school entry, enjoy better language and mathematical skills, demon-strate fewer problem behaviours, and form better peer relationships than children in poorer-quality centres when assessed at the end of second grade. These CQO results are consistent with those reported by studies conducted in Canada (E.V. Jacobs, Selig, and White 1992) and Sweden (Broberg et al. 1997).

Higher-quality care is associated with better developmental outcomes for children across the socioeconomic spectrum of family circumstances (Peisner-Feinberg et al. 1999, 10). However, findings from the Perry Pre-school Program (Berrueta-Clement et al. 1984), which targeted children from at-risk households, suggest that participation in quality child care is especially beneficial for children from families with low socioeco-nomic status. The cost-benefit analysis of this program indicates that, "over the lifetimes of the participants, preschool is estimated to yield economic benefits with an estimated present value that is over seven times the cost of one year of the program" (1). Similar results were found recently in New York City. An evaluation of the Abecedarian Early Child-hood Intervention for very young low-income children estimates a cost-benefit ratio of $4 return for every $1 of investment in the program (Masse and Barnett 2002).

Labour Supply
Not only can quality child care factor positively in human-capital for-mation among future workers, but it can also influence labour supply. Population aging is a reality that governments must grapple with cross-nationally. In Canada, the warped population pyramid will reduce la-bour supply in the absence of a dramatic increase in immigration. Denton and Spencer (1999, Figure 4) estimate that labour force growth rates will drop from roughly 6 percent in 2001 to below 2 percent by 2011 and fall to nearly zero thereafter until 2031.

Deferring retirement among citizens over fifty-five is the remedy to anticipated labour shortages that receives the most attention in the literature (for example, Denton and Spencer 1999, 10-13). But postponing retirement is just one piece of the puzzle. Fertility also merits attention, as Canada has witnessed a declining birth rate since 1960. In 1997 there were just forty-four births for every thousand women aged fifteen to forty-nine, less than half the birth rate in 1959, and 23 percent lower than in 1990 (Statistics Canada 2000, 34). The declining birth rate is directly related to growing work-life conflict. In their most recent study of work-life balance among employees of large firms, Duxbury and Higgins (2003, 40) report that "approximately one in five Canadians have decided to limit their family size in an attempt to deal with the issues associated with work and family." A slightly larger share of people also delay starting a family due to job demands. Quebeckers, who report the highest levels of work-family balance in the country, are the least likely to delay having children (41). The fact that this province is the only jurisdiction in the country to be instituting a universal system of child care is likely no coincidence.

The correlation between work-family balance and fertility in Quebec is borne out in the international arena. Until the 1970s, Organisation for Economic Co-operation and Development (OECD) data reveal, fertility was negatively related to the level of women's labour force participation (1999, 16). The inverse is now true (ibid.). Family size is lowest in countries where women's labour force participation rate is weakest. While the OECD is careful to acknowledge that "such simple comparisons do not prove that increasing female labour force participation will inevitably increase fertility rates, they do suggest that child-rearing and paid work are *complementary*, rather than *alternative* activities" (ibid.).

The positive relationship between women's attainment of work-life balance and fertility is further confirmed by the Scandinavian experience. Empowered by generous employment leave and child care benefits, Nordic countries managed to reverse the fertility decline in the 1980s while their European neighbours did not. As Esping-Andersen (2002, 65-66) observes,

> beginning in the 1960s-1970s, we see everywhere a steady fall in birth rates, hitting all time lows (1.4) in Northern Europe in the late 1970s, a little later elsewhere. The great international bifurcation begins at this point. One group of countries, mainly the Scandinavian, experience a resurgence of fertility in tandem with women's employment; most other European countries remain caught in a low fertility equilibrium even if

female participation remains low. Most telling is the sharp drop in Swedish fertility during the 1990s, which coincides with a 7 percentage point decline in female employment. The core issue, obviously, has to do with how women succeed in combining paid work and children.

Although higher birth rates encouraged by work-family balance policy have the potential to increase labour supply, any effect of renewed fertility on labour force growth will be delayed at least two decades as children are nurtured to become active labour market participants. A relative shortage of labour is thus a reality in Canada and in other affluent nations for many years, regardless of the reproductive decisions its citizens make today. The search for labour in the near term will need to occur elsewhere.

One theme that is underexamined in Canadian literature is the effect that limited labour force growth will have on women's employment. Historically, the ideology of motherhood has been malleable to the demands of capitalism, as was particularly evident during the war years. When industry required additional labour to fill positions vacated by male soldiers, women were welcomed into the labour market by firms and governments alike. As discussed earlier, the federal government went so far as to introduce the intergovernmental Day Nurseries Agreements to subsidize child care for mothers.

Population aging is re-creating a tighter labour environment. Just as the war-induced shortage of labour in the 1940s propelled many women into war industries and related occupations, so the echo of the postwar baby boom is likely to motivate employers to draw on the (albeit much smaller) reserve pool of labour that some women continue to represent. In particular, coaxing mothers to shift from part-time to full-time hours may be one strategy that firms and governments employ to sustain labour supply and tax revenue as the share of older citizens grows. Since young women are now more likely than their male counterparts to earn a university degree (Statistics Canada 2000, 86), this female cohort is bound to appear as an especially attractive source of human capital. The cost of child care, however, will be a critical factor in determining the extent to which firms can count on accessing this capital. Research by Powell (1997), for instance, shows that the hours of paid work that Canadian mothers perform is directly influenced by child care fees: a 10 percent decrease in the cost of care can be expected to increase maternal employment time by over 3 percent. The care*fair* recommendation that Canadian governments collaborate to create a child care system that would reduce parent fees to roughly 20 percent of the total cost of care would, therefore, have dramatic positive consequences for maternal labour supply at the very moment when the country must grapple with the challenges posed by stagnant labour force growth.

Time Crunch

The dramatic increase in female labour force participation has resulted in a time squeeze for households. Men and women encounter a modern time crunch because they are less likely to benefit from having someone at home who is devoted to domestic activity (J.A. Jacobs and Gerson 2000, 100). In liberal welfare regimes, market hours are rising more than non-market time is declining when measured at the household level – a trend that affects the total paid and unpaid work schedules of women disproportionately compared to men. This trend will be exacerbated if firms aim to attract additional paid worktime from women to compensate for slower labour force growth.

It is a mistake to assume contemporary households perform additional paid work hours simply to indulge in new levels of consumerism that were not evident three decades ago. The US example is instructive on this point, since that country is the front-runner in terms of average paid work hours performed per working-age citizen. Bluestone and Rose (2000, 30) report that the typical American dual-earner family enjoyed only a modest 18.5 percent increase in real earnings between 1973 and 1988 as a result of a 16.3 percent increase in paid hours. When the data is disaggregated by educational attainment, the story is more telling still:

> For all families – with the notable exception of those headed by a worker with at least a college degree – the enormous increase in work effort over the past twenty years has accomplished no more than permit families to maintain their *old* standard of living. For high school drop-out families, the situation has been even tougher. Between 1973 and 1988, these families increased their annual work effort by nearly 12 per cent yet ended up with 8 per cent *less* annual income. For families headed by high school graduates or some college, work effort was up by 16-17.4 per cent. All of these added hours of work left such families with less than a 4 per cent increase in total earnings. These families are trapped in an Alice in Wonderland world, running faster and faster just to stay in the same place. (30-31)

In Canada, the Alice in Wonderland phenomenon is undermining the levels of well-being that labour force participants report. According to the Duxbury and Higgins (2003, 34) sample, 58 percent of employees "are currently experiencing high levels of role overload (i.e. have too much to do in a given amount of time)." This figure is up 20 percentage points since the last decade. The Duxbury and Higgins findings also indicate that the costs of role overload are borne particularly in the domestic sphere. Work obligations far more regularly interfere with Canadians' abilities to fulfill their responsibilities at home than vice versa (35). The result is that the majority of Canadian families report they are not satisfied or are only moderately satisfied with the way their family deals with conflicts, spends its leisure time, and communicates with household members (38-39). Not surprisingly, employed Canadians with dependent care responsibilities are the most likely to report less control over their time and problems balancing work and family (35).

Despite his stated interest in family policy, Esping-Andersen does not examine measures that would provide citizens with more time out of the labour force. This is somewhat ironic given that the concept of decommodification drives his original welfare regime typology. It is also surprising, since he acknowledges that "a hallmark of new, emerging family forms is that they suffer from a scarcity of time" (1999, 57). However, Esping-Andersen's interest in time-strapped homes pertains principally to their potential to function as an engine of employment growth. With the clarity that is characteristic of his work, he observes that publicly supporting dual-earner families with substantial investment in child care services will, in turn, accelerate demand for other services. As he puts it,

> universalizing the double earning household (with lots of children) holds yet another promise of welfare improvement. When we add its greater purchasing power to its desperate search for free time, it is a truly promising source of service consumption, from restaurants and leisure parks to child care and home-help services for their aged parents. Thereby families create jobs for waiters, park-keepers, child-minders, and home-helpers. Of course, access to child care is a pre-condition for dual-income families in the first place. This is exactly the point: services beget services; the double-earner household plays the role of employment multiplier. (179)

Esping-Andersen's recognition of the employment-creation potential inherent in time-strapped households is insightful, and it provides additional support for the sort of child care recommendations I defend in the previous chapter. But his discussion also completely ignores the harm that can accompany overextension in the labour market. Citizens are not just concerned about their level of income; they are also concerned about the amount of time they must spend to earn it, since long hours in the labour force mean sacrificing participation in other important areas of social life (see also Osberg 2001).

One strength of the care*fair* reform package outlined in this book is that it defends against this weakness of Esping-Andersen's third way model. It acknowledges that time in domesticity is a necessary condition for social belonging. The proposed reforms to employment leave and labour standards regulating hours of paid work aim directly to provide more of this time for diverse groups of women and men, while simultaneously challenging the gender division of care. Swedish experience foreshadows the efficacy of the employment leave provisions. Although the country's comprehensive system of public child care means that Swedish rates of female labour force participation exceed those in the United States, the Swedish parental leave system also gives parents the opportunity to care personally and exclusively for their children until their first birthday. The result is that, during the early 1990s, 95 percent of Swedish infants were in parental care alone, whereas this was the case for just a bare majority of American infants (Sainsbury 1996, 100). Denmark, in turn, has recently succeeded in implementing employment practices that see the majority of full-time workers of both genders performing usual paid workweeks of between thirty-six and thirty-seven hours (Mutari and Figart 2001, 48). This shift toward shorter full-time workweeks for both men and women is well on the way to the thirty-five-hour norm that care*fair* prescribes.

In the final sections of this chapter, I develop the discussion of employment leave and standards regulating paid work hours in a different direction, in order to provide further justification to revise full-time work norms. In addition to their ability to tackle gender inequality and time poverty, I argue that care*fair* measures include resources to address some of the inequalities that have emerged as a result of the recent polarization of paid worktime. Specifically, measures designed to promote non-market time at a societal level can be expected to contribute modestly to the provision of additional earning opportunities for individual citizens who presently suffer too few hours in the market.

Earnings Inequality and Un(der)employment
The polarization of paid work hours that widened the divide between core and periphery labour force participants in Canada has increased market earnings inequality. Between 1981 and 1989, weekly earnings

inequality grew 13 percent among Canadian male workers and 5 percent among women labour force participants (Morissette, Myles, and Picot 1995, 37). The rise in inequality among men was driven by two factors: (i) growing inequality in the distribution of paid work hours; and (ii) changing work patterns among low- and high-wage labour force participants, which saw the latter group assume longer hours more regularly than the former. Earnings inequality grew more slowly among women workers because there was less inequality in the distribution of worktime. As more women moved from standard hours to long workweeks, more part-time women employees also put in longer hours. Thus, the more modest growth in earnings inequality among women was due entirely to the second factor affecting men: relative to low-wage workers, a greater share of higher-paid women worked long workweeks in 1989 than in 1981 (38). Since the late 1980s, data indicate that earnings inequality has levelled off for both sexes (Picot 1998).

One implication of the finding that the distribution of paid worktime powered the polarization of earnings is that policies which target wage levels alone will be insufficient to remedy the earnings inequality that has been entrenched since 1989. Wage levels do not address the shortage of paid hours that accounts significantly for falling earnings in the bottom income deciles. To reverse this trend, policy makers must reduce the incentives that disincline companies to hire additional workers or redistribute job responsibilities between a larger number of employees (Morissette, Myles, and Picot 1995, 44). The proposed reduction of standard work hours to increase the cost of weekly labour over thirty-five hours (averaged over a year) is one important step toward changing this incentive structure. Legislators could further refine incentives by converting some labour expenses that are currently fixed into costs that would vary according to hours of work. For instance, Morissette, Myles, and Picot (1995, 44) observe that payroll taxes for programs like the C/QPP, EI, and employer contributions for fringe benefits typically reach a maximum when employee earnings rise above a specified level. As a result, it is advantageous for employers to retain higher-paid workers for longer hours instead of hiring additional workers to increase output when their business requires firm-specific skills and absorbs training costs. In place of the current system, which calculates employer contributions based entirely on employee income, new policies could base payroll taxes partially in terms of an employee's hours. Rates could increase linearly or progressively, with the outcome that employers incur added costs for overtime employment.

The distribution of paid worktime that drove rising earnings inequality in the 1980s in Canada is symptomatic of broader problems of persistent unemployment domestically and internationally. In response, in some European countries the concept of worksharing has represented the hope (and sometimes conviction) that a reduction in hours per full-time worker will spread the available demand for labour more broadly and thereby increase aggregate employment (see J. Hunt 1998, 339). This hope represented the primary motivation behind the worktime redistribution plans implemented in France and Germany over the past two decades.

The most recent economic research reveals that worksharing is not a primary solution to problems of persistent unemployment. In a review of job growth created by European government interventions designed to redistribute paid worktime, Freeman (1998, 196) concludes that, "while worksharing can increase employment, most government-sponsored efforts to spread work have had limited efficacy." The countries that tried worksharing in the past two decades to mitigate rising unemployment already had low levels of normal worktime. Since extant work practices provided these countries with limited room to innovate, Freeman posits that worksharing may be more successful in economies in which full-time employees typically work longer hours, such as in Spain, Japan, the United States, or Canada (210). Still, the relative lack of success in Europe provides little reason to believe that other states can attain results that are significantly more successful. This view is now the consensus, held even by those who initially expected worksharing to sharply reduce unemployment (ibid., note 14).

Economists measure the employment effects of worksharing in terms of the number of jobs generated or lost relative to the size of the reduction in paid working hours (the elasticity of jobs to hours). Freeman's (1998, 207-10) review of existing literature suggests that worktime reductions in Europe all had positive (although small) effects for employment, reporting elasticity coefficients that range from 0.08 to 0.4. This range indicates that a 10 percent reduction in paid hours can be expected to generate an increase in employment of somewhere between 0.8 percent and 4 percent. Huberman and Lanoie (2000, 144) support Freeman's finding, reporting that international studies indicate elasticities of jobs to hours that range from 0.3 to 0.8. They also add to the existing body of research by examining worksharing initiatives implemented by four corporations and one provincial government ministry in Quebec in the 1990s: the elasticities found in these employment contexts ranged from 0.14 to 0.68 (146). Similarly, Bosch (1993, 147) summarizes the findings of roughly a dozen German worksharing studies, all of which "conclude that working-time reductions had a positive employment effect." The elasticity of jobs to employment in these cases ranged from 0.4 to 0.75.

Although not a primary solution to persistent un(der)employment, these data reflect the broad consensus in the worksharing literature that worktime redistribution will at least not exacerbate unemployment levels and is more likely to generate positive, albeit very modest, employment gains. Given the importance of employment for dignified community membership suggested by neoliberals, third way proponents, and feminists, the possibility of generating even moderate increases in job openings as a result of measures designed to promote gender equality is further justification for the policy shifts recommended in Chapter 7.

Of particular interest is the fact that research indicates that extended blocks of time off – such as paid leave arrangements, career breaks, or early retirement – offer the most potential for job creation through worksharing (Advisory Group 1994, 60; Freeman 1998, 209). Studies suggest that technological processes and cost structures are such that firms are more likely to replace an incumbent worker who leaves the firm temporarily (or permanently in the case of early retirement) with a new employee than they are to respond to a statutory reduction in standard full-time hours by hiring additional labour. This finding provides added reason to reconsider public financial commitments to parental leave, calculating its cost in reference to the potential EI and social assistance savings that can be expected from extended leave periods. Canadian policy makers may also wish to follow one element of the Spanish leave system to further capitalize on the potential employment gains implicit in parental leave policy. Since 1998, employers in Spain have been exempt from paying social security contributions for the contracts of workers recruited to replace those on leave for maternity, adoption, or foster parenting (European Industrial Relations Review 2001b, 14).

Given the job-growth potential that resides in employment leave schemes, Canadian governments have reason to consider leave measures that extend beyond maternity and parental benefits. The Danish government has recently experimented on this front, instituting a system of subsidized leave that supplements the country's regular parental insurance system. In the mid-1990s, all Danish employees became eligible to take educational, caregiving, and personal sabbatical leaves of up to one year, conditional on the agreement of their employers. While on leave, employees could claim unemployment insurance: 100 percent of regular benefits for educational leave and 60 percent for caregiving and personal leave.

The personal sabbatical option of the Danish program is especially innovative and unique. It permits citizens to take a leave of absence for any purpose, provided that the company hires an unemployed person as a replacement. In effect, the sabbatical functions as an exchange of wages and unemployment benefits between someone with and someone without a job. The system provides Danish citizens with added flexibility to balance not only unpaid child, dependent, and elder care, but also other important citizenry pursuits, with employment throughout the life course. The possible savings to government make this option attractive, since the program has the potential to swap full EI benefits paid to a jobless person in favour of 60 percent of benefits paid to a person on leave.

Before emulating such a program, however, it will be important for Canadian governments to learn from mistakes in Denmark. Siim (1998, 386) reports that the leave system "created 'bottle-necks,' because the leave-takers are concentrated in a few occupations." Leaves are particularly common among women in the public sector, including nurses. The specialized training required of nurses did not allow them to be replaced easily, with the result that the country faced a shortage of nurses. In low-skilled positions, job-swap rates were also relatively low, in part because of the structure of employment standards. The leave program awarded the worker on sabbatical the right to keep her or his position in the company, while laws of job tenure made it difficult to dismiss new workers. Employers were understandably reluctant to hire replacement staff if it meant they might end up paying salaries to two people to do the job of one (Cox 1998, 403). Finally, Danish leave benefits were also available to the unemployed. This design feature diminished the positive labour market effects of the policy, since the leave schemes provided a socially sanctioned alternative to the status of unemployment (Siim 1998, 386).

While research indicates that employment leave schemes have modest job growth potential, J. Hunt (1999) expresses skepticism about earlier studies that report positive employment effects from reducing standard workweeks, particularly in Germany. She points out that most of the German evaluations consist of either surveys of firms before and after worksharing policies were introduced, or econometric studies that rely on aggregate time series data. In both approaches, the effect of falling standard hours could be confounded with the effects of other factors. To avoid this methodological problem, she takes advantage of industry-level variation in standard-hours reductions in West Germany to evaluate the impact of working-time transitions on employment. Her results suggest that reductions in standard hours actually caused very small employment losses among German men. The reason for the decline in employment, she argues, is that actual reductions in hours were not accompanied by an associated drop in income. The result was a de facto wage increase, which renders unlikely the possibility of an employment rise in response to reduced standard hours, since labour is more expensive. However, her analysis also acknowledges the possibility of increased employment through other worksharing strategies that do not require firms to compensate employees fully for lost hours of work.

Given the risk of employment losses if worksharing requires firms to compensate workers fully for reduced hours, proponents of worktime redistribution to promote gender equality must countenance the reality that some workers stand to endure declines in real earnings. One result of the diminishing fortunes of recent market entrants is a generation of male workers who are more likely to resist the redistribution of paid worktime on the grounds that they are less able to afford the loss of income associated with fewer working hours. Accordingly, Huberman and Lanoie (2000, 152) suggest that the success of worktime redistribution in Canada depends importantly on transitional government incentives designed to minimize the wage penalty associated with working less. Huberman and Lanoie examine various case studies, including one that shows the company Alcan enjoyed the most significant positive employment effect, largely because employees' earnings losses from worktime reductions were mitigated by federal and provincial wage subsidies (149). The cost-benefit analysis developed by Lanoie and Raymond (1999) shows that the federal subsidy was more than offset by the reduction in EI payments that would have been issued. The benefits to the provincial government were less obvious, however, since the same study found limited change in provincial welfare expenditures as a result of the firm's increase in jobs.

In addition to transitional incentives, enriched child care and parental leave benefits could also provide the basis for broader societal commitments to wage moderation. Such commitments are important for the long-term success of worktime redistribution, since demand for employment will be more robust as the cost of labour becomes more competitive relative to the cost of capital. By supplementing income substantially when private financial pressures grow especially acute, child care and parental leave benefits hold some potential to mitigate citizens' concerns about trading wage increases for a reduction in paid working hours, at least among the 80-plus percent of Canadians who become parents.

There is precedent in Canada for using family benefits as wage-restraint measures. The federal government implemented universal family allowances in 1945, in large part to promote economic stabilization goals. The finance department intended the family allowance plan to mitigate labour demands for higher wages following years of wartime restraint (Ursel 1992, 190-98). A care*fair* agenda would see Canada revisit this sort of wage moderation strategy. In return for added care*fair* benefits (and additional time for family and leisure), citizens would acknowledge an obligation to dampen wage demands. Explicit in this obligation would be the expectation that citizens recognize the social value generated when individuals take future productivity gains in the form of reduced worktime so that the benefits of economic growth can be shared among more workers in a manner that challenges systemic barriers to gender equality.

9
From LEGO™ to Teeter-Totter: Social Investment in Work-Life Balance

The sort of child-centred social investment state that Esping-Andersen (2002, Chapter 2) outlines has been dubbed the LEGO™ model by Jenson (2003). The LEGO™ metaphor distinguishes this third way vision from the neoliberal trampoline ideal of restricting the scope of state insurance so that citizens bounce back to the market or family in search of security. It also differentiates the social investment state from the postwar social liberal safety net ideal that sought to create a system of social protection that would insure citizens during periods when they could not make their livelihood through market participation alone.

Jenson maintains that, given LEGO™ branding, her label aptly captures the tenor of the social investment state. The toy building-block company sees "children as natural learners. These are precious qualities that should be nurtured and stimulated throughout life ... 'Play' in the LEGO sense is learning. By helping children to learn, we build confident, curious and resourceful adults. For their future. And ours" (http://www.lego.com/build in Jenson 2003, 17-18).

This element of the company's philosophy illustrates three fundamental features of the social investment state (Jenson 2003, 18). The third way vision focuses on lifelong learning, as does LEGO™. Child's play, for the third way, is socially valuable when it is educationally stimulating; it excites and fosters the capacity for continuous learning and thus prepares children for their adult working years when they will need to adapt flexibly to the new social risks and opportunities that the knowledge economy represents. The third way vision further acknowledges that social investment in individuals, especially in children, is in the interest of society as a whole, just as the LEGO™ corporation suggests that the childhood play which prepares children for their working years will have benefits that spill over to society – "For their future. And ours."

The ideal of the social investment state also employs the same life-course perspective that is evident in the LEGO™ philosophy. The third way vision is future oriented; it emphasizes equality of opportunity over the entire life course more than static equality of consumption. This precept underpins Esping-Andersen's (1999, 182) interest in a "mobility guarantee" to prevent lifelong entrapment in the low-wage work that is a reality of the postindustrial economy. As he puts it, "what we are trying to resolve is a dynamic, life course issue and not where to place everybody today. A new welfare optimum is, in fact, compatible with the possibility that many of us will experience a spell of unpleasant-ness" (183; see also Giddens 1999, 101). The challenge confronting the social investment state, therefore, is to institute a system of prevention that ensures periodic hardship is temporary and not long term. Poverty traps, particularly in the early years, are problematic because they com-promise citizens' futures.

The care*fair* reforms proposed in this book are sympathetic to the third way insights that the LEGO™ model represents. But, alone, the LEGO™ metaphor is inadequate as a vision for postindustrial welfare. It focuses too much on work.

Third way academics such as Esping-Andersen and Giddens are quick to concede that this work focus is problematic if it entirely erodes com-mitment to more traditional social insurance measures. Giddens (1999, 110) acknowledges that our vision of inclusion "must stretch well be-yond work," in large part "because there are many people at any one time not able to be in the labour force," especially so long as economies suffer structural unemployment. Analysis of work-poor households moves Esping-Andersen (2002, 39) to a similar conclusion: "An exaggerated bias in favour of 'make-work-pay' policy has substantial risks," he maintains. His calculations suggest that more than half of workless households in Europe include the chronically ill, the disabled, and women who have never held a job. These social groups represent what he terms the "hard-core" excluded, for whom integration in the labour market is not a vi-able social security strategy (43). In his international review of active labour market policy, he also finds that just one-third of cases represent clear successes in which individuals fully escape from welfare depend-ency; a second third enjoys only a partial or temporary reprieve; the final third remains fully dependent (49). The implication is that passive social insurance measures will remain a necessity in any postindustrial welfare regime concerned with social security and justice.

Despite this third way concession, the life-course employment focus that motivates the LEGO™ model remains incomplete. A social vision too engrossed with the work ethic represents an impoverished, unattractive ideal that neglects the diversity of goals that life has to offer, including family and other meaningful relationships that emerge principally outside of market contexts. Giddens acknowledges this theme rhetorically (1999, 110), but he does not integrate it fully into the social investment state architecture he describes. The same problem inflicts the work of Esping-Andersen. Absent in the third way ideal at present is any concerted effort to embrace and make time for relationships that define our lives as parents, kin, friends, lovers, or neighbours.

Therefore, in place of LEGO™, I think a more appropriate metaphor for postindustrial welfare is the teeter-totter. Like LEGO™, this children's playground toy evokes a life-course focus that recognizes the importance of the early years and the benefits that accrue to society from social investments in childhood. But the teeter-totter also conveys the dynamic image of a balancing act and, as such, is an appropriate metaphor for integrating paid work with family and other non-labour-market pursuits. The up-and-down movement of the teeter-totter conveys the ebb and flow of the life course: at some stages our time is more weighted with family responsibilities; at other moments the balance must shift so that earning and career aspirations can ascend in priority. The to-and-fro continues to interweave various personal pursuits with the necessity of income generation until we make a final retreat from the labour force as seniors.

The teeter-totter metaphor can also reflect the reality that some citizens will suffer periods of undesired unemployment, much as a slim child can be stranded mid-air by her heavier playmate at the opposite end of the teeter-totter. As on the supervised playground, the appropriate response includes both protection and guidance: protection in the guise of financial assistance to tide over the out-of-work; and guidance in the form of publicly provided and (if need be) imposed suggestions about how to escape the predicament and get down to work again.

While the teeter-totter permits participants playful opportunities to strike a balancing act that suits their respective personal preferences – the activity may be bumpy or gentle, evenly paced or off-beat – no one seat on the toy stays grounded permanently. Teeter-tottering is all about give and take, about reciprocity. The metaphor therefore captures the expectation of reciprocity that care*fair* demands of men when it comes to distributing care work. There is no room on the teeter-totter for free riders. All participants must exert themselves to ensure both ends of the playground toy rise and fall.

The teeter-totter metaphor will leave many political thinkers in unfamiliar territory. Nurturing or enjoying familial and other relationships is a sphere of activity that Western philosophical traditions which contemplate the good life have largely overlooked (see also Walzer 1991). The civic republican tradition, we have seen, argues that to live well is to be politically active in the public sphere. The Marxist responds that the life we should aspire toward is that of the renaissance producer: one who interweaves artistry, invention, and craftsmanship. The libertarian/neoliberal good life rejects these two answers to depict citizens as consumers in the market. It is not a question of political involvement or what we produce that determines a life well lived. The act of making choices, whatever they favour, is what is most important for the libertarian, and markets free from all but the most modest state interference best permit the necessary autonomy. Those with communitarian or social conservative inclinations have still another take, which is cautious about the amorality and disloyalty that market consumerism risks fostering. They argue, instead, that the preferred setting for the good life is the community, in which we are bound to one another by ties of blood, history, and/or shared values.

The communitarian vision comes closest to acknowledging the importance of relationships for individual well-being in terms of material and emotional security, as well as identity and belonging. But the ties of blood and history that historically have interested the communitarian tradition are most often those of the ethnic group, rather than the relations of family or domesticity with which I am concerned. What is more, the communitarian ideal suffers a single-mindedness that plagues all four philosophical traditions. The reality of the postindustrial world means it is naïve to think any one of the above four answers captures all there is to say about the good life. This is Walzer's (1991, 298) point when he argues that civil society is the most supportive environment for the good life because civil society is a "setting of settings": it is the diverse "ground where all versions of the good are worked out and tested ... and proved to be partial [and] incomplete." The fact is that a life well lived today is bound to include elements from all four traditions – political activity, production, consumerism, and community membership – as well as practices that these traditions largely neglect. I have argued that time for domestic activities is one area that has been ignored too long, since developing caring relationships is an integral thread in almost everyone's tapestry of life projects.

Because our philosophical traditions have largely discounted the private time that is necessary for social inclusion, it is important to return to T.H. Marshall's (1964, 104) insight about what determines the qualitative content of social rights and obligations in any society. "Expectations officially recognized as legitimate," he reminds us, "become, as it were, details in a design for community living." The argument implicit throughout this book is that work-family balance (as promoted by the recommended care*fair* reforms) is, and should be acknowledged as, a legitimate citizenry expectation. The expectation draws legitimacy from normative, practical, strategic, and ideological considerations.

A more robust public commitment to facilitate work-family balance is important for normative reasons because it would address the three pillars of social citizenship that Marshall (1964) and Rawls (1971) identify in their formative work on the subject: social security, substantive equality of opportunity, and full inclusion across important areas of community life. Personal security in the postindustrial economy demands that citizens acquire sufficient levels of human capital to succeed and adapt in the dynamic labour force in which knowledge is an increasingly important commodity. Economic conservatives, third way advocates, and feminists who work in the tradition of Pateman (1989) support this characterization of security by emphasizing the welfare potential of market participation, particularly for minimizing dependency. The first half of the work-family balance concept captures this shared insight, indicating concern to counter systemic barriers to employment for some social groups, while also prioritizing education and retraining to offset structural unemployment and any mismatch between the skills demanded by employers and those possessed by the un(der)employed.

By contrast, the second half of the work-family balance concept acknowledges that one's private sphere of intimate relations is also an important source of welfare that state social services cannot replace. Families that function well have the potential to provide their members with emotional and material resources, often in a dignified manner that other institutions can rarely match. The early postwar paradigm explicitly capitalized on this reality by institutionalizing distinct citizenship roles for economically and racially privileged women to provide welfare in the domestic sphere. The social and economic costs for women associated with this fragmented and marginalized citizenry role are problematic, as has been discussed throughout the book. But the costs do not mean the work is any less significant for individual security or that citizens do not have a responsibility, and in many cases a genuine desire, to care and nurture in domestic contexts in order to foster the autonomy of intimate relations. Feminists, communitarians, and social conservatives all acknowledge citizenry responsibilities and aspirations to care privately, although the schools of thought diverge over the question of men's obligations.

The issue of male citizenry duties, however, is fundamental to societal commitments to substantive equality of opportunity. Equality of opportunity implies not only that individuals will be evaluated strictly on the basis of their qualifications for positions, but also, and more fundamentally, that individuals should have the same chances to acquire the qualifications for desirable positions. Throughout the book, I have argued that the latter requirement of equal opportunity is not simply a matter of the distribution of material resources. The distribution of roles and responsibilities is just as important. Specifically, the persistent hegemony of the female caregiver model constrains the time and opportunities available to women to labour in the paid workforce and acquire the level of human capital associated with financial security and occupational advancement. In response, the theme of work-family balance signals a strategy by which to remedy the present distribution of responsibility for caregiving. It illuminates the need to make paid work and unpaid care more compatible in order to give some women new opportunities to pursue success in the labour market, while also facilitating (and demanding) that more men assume greater responsibility for care work so as to restructure the existing gender order.

Although a work-family balance framework expresses concern to equalize employment-related opportunities between the sexes, it resists a one-dimensional workerist understanding of social inclusion. The latter half of the balancing act heightens public awareness about the value of participation in one's sphere of personal relations and the legitimacy of individual desires to spend more time there. Therefore, under the concept of work-family balance, equality of opportunity implies minimizing social and economic factors that limit the time some citizens can afford to spend among intimate relations, in addition to mitigating barriers that impede access to the public spaces of market and political arena. This equal-opportunity commitment motivates renewed concern for decommodifying social programs that may be especially important to some lower-income and single women for whom financial necessity impedes the fulfillment of their desires to nurture and care at home. Decommodifying measures that render more domestic time affordable will also be important for giving some men the incentive to redefine their present roles as secondary carers.

The intention to equalize domestic opportunities implicit in the work-family balance concept signals a fundamental insight about community membership that has been neglected by liberal understandings of citizenship, which prioritize inclusion in public domains. The latter half of the work-family balance concept suggests that our understanding of full community membership is impoverished if it takes the private sphere for granted or views it only in instrumentalist terms. Following feminists who contribute to the literature associated with Collins (1991, 1994), the alternative framework urges the state to regard the private sphere of spousal, family, and friendship relationships as a vital site of citizenry activity that can protect individuals from isolation, foster and redefine personal identity, validate one's sense of self-worth, provide a reprieve from discriminatory social forces, and empower individuals and the diverse communities in which they belong. In response to this recognition, the work-family balance metaphor points to the importance of building a social policy blueprint that integrates the need for private unpaid time into broader institutional planning.

Although it elevates participation in the domestic sphere to the same status as inclusion in the market and political arena, the work-family balance concept fully acknowledges the insights linking paid work with dignified social inclusion that are advanced by third way proponents, economic conservatives, and feminists who work in the tradition of Pateman (1989). Under neoliberalism, performance of paid work emerged as the primary social duty, in return for which one earns entitlement to social security. But significantly higher rates of unemployment over the past twenty-five years compared to the first postwar decades indicate that the postindustrial transition has eroded the context in which individuals seeking paid work can claim sufficient time in the labour market as a right of citizenship. In response, a work-family balance framework acknowledges that the distribution of paid and unpaid time is a matter of distributive justice that is importantly influenced by state regulations governing employment standards and industrial relations, monetary and taxation policies, and social expenditure. The framework therefore prioritizes public policy changes to redefine cultural constructs of full-time employment. Restructuring the existing gender order is the primary goal of this policy trajectory because it would render paid work and unpaid caregiving more compatible. However, a further implication of the policy shift is a modest potential to redistribute paid worktime between the employed and the un(der)employed in order to foster increased opportunities for genuine social inclusion among the latter.

Since enhanced public commitments to work-family balance would contribute importantly to promoting security, substantive equality, and full participation across important areas of social life, citizens have solid normative grounds on which to demand reorganization of the public sphere to better accommodate this balancing act. But in addition to questions of distributive justice, there are also significant practical factors that motivate this state restructuring. The postindustrial transition has meant declining real wages for men, as well as income and job polarization. These structural shifts intersected ideological changes that powered the transition from the so-called traditional family of the first postwar decades, one result of which is considerably higher rates of female labour force participation. Together, the two broad socioeconomic transitions mean that most families can no longer financially afford, nor necessarily desire, to have one partner remain home to specialize in unpaid domestic work. This option is even more remote for most of the rising number of single-parent families. The resultant shift within households away from unpaid domestic time in favour of increased paid time means that families increasingly encounter a time crunch. As households adapt their planning strategies to resist the financial squeeze that became more common for many Canadians during most of the 1990s, one significant opportunity cost is lost leisure and less time with partners, children, friends, and the broader community. Lost unpaid time disrupts collective time rhythms and augments stress. Single mothers and married mothers who work full-time are particularly prone to higher levels of stress and the related health ailments.

A work-family balance framework for social citizenship would partially address the growing time poverty that citizens endure on two fronts. First, the stress encountered by parents who struggle to find suitable care arrangements for children while on the job would be minimized by instituting quality child care programs that are affordable for all families. Second, the framework would institutionalize new, affordable opportunities for unpaid time by implementing enriched subsidized employment leave benefits, and would encourage citizens to share in future productivity gains in the form of time away from paid work.

Work-family balance is also a legitimate expectation for strategic reasons, insofar as the concept includes resources to address multiple social problems simultaneously. As already discussed, redefining cultural constructs of full-time employment is expected to generate modest employment gains. The same policy measures have the capacity to mitigate earnings polarization. Research indicates that policies which target wage levels alone will prove insufficient to stabilize the earnings of those in the bottom income deciles, since a shortage of paid hours accounts significantly for their falling income. The care*fair* framework would address this finding by reducing incentives that disincline companies to hire additional workers or redistribute job tasks between a larger number of employees, all as part of the broader goal to render unpaid work and paid employment more compatible. Enriched child care and parental leave entitlements also have some potential to mitigate poverty among families with young children, which has grown more common over the past two decades, in part because of declining real wages for men. Both public benefits would respond to citizens' financial pressures during life-course periods when private expenses are particularly high and income is often relatively low. Child care facilitates continued labour force participation and reduces the cost of alternative care arrangements, while enriched parental leave would enable more parents (including fathers) to remain home with young children to avoid the substantial expense of non-parental care.

Finally, the expectation of work-family balance is legitimate in the contemporary setting for ideological reasons. The neoliberal discourse that rose to prominence in the past two decades favours the individual responsibility model of the family, which presumes that single citizens should be capable of shouldering both the earning and the caregiving roles. This assumption underpins the economic conservative interest in extending work duties to mothers to minimize social assistance caseloads, while simultaneously reducing government commitments to care-related social services, as is the practice currently in British Columbia. A care*fair* framework for social citizenship would retain the neoliberal idea that the social citizen is one who can balance adequate participation in private and public spaces, but would reverse the policy course in which neoliberals privatized many welfare services to the domestic and voluntary sector. This reversal is necessary if we are to ensure that the act of balancing work and family is not just a rhetorical ideal, but is also a realistic possibility for most in society.

Neoliberal ideology also primes citizens of liberal welfare regimes to link entitlement to social benefits with the discharge of social duties. The care*fair* reforms proposed in this book would extend the sympathy for welfare contractualism that already defines our cultural context so that its principle of reciprocity embraces caregiving responsibilities and rights. The emergence of workfare signals heightened contempt for free riding on social insurance. It is therefore culturally legitimate for citizens to expect governments now to demonstrate a similar contempt for the free ride on female care that underpins men's patriarchal dividend.

Notes

Chapter 2: The American Express™ Model of Citizenship

1 Rawls's presumption about agency raises important ontological questions. Most notably, Sandel (1984, 86) remarks that the original position implies that "no role or commitment could define me so completely that I could not understand myself without it. No project could be so essential that turning away from it would call into question the person I am." This ontological implication merits careful scrutiny, something Sandel pursues in "The Procedural Republic and the Unencumbered Self" (1984). See Kymlicka (1989) for an alternative perspective.

Chapter 3: The Celebrated Idiot

1 Stan Rogers, "The Idiot." On *Northwest Passage* (Dundas, ON: Fogarty's Cove Music, 1981).

Chapter 4: The Idiot's Acumen

1 *Order in Council authorizing agreements with provinces for the care of children whose mothers or foster mothers are employed in war industries in Canada*, P.C. 1942-6242.

Chapter 7: Care*fair*

1 Budget Implementation Act, 2000, S.C. 2000, c. 14. Section 3(2) extended the duration of parental leave benefits from ten to thirty-five weeks.
2 I am indebted to Professor Anita Nyberg for providing the parental leave data from Sweden. She works at Svensk modell i förändring Arbetslivsinstitutet, 112 79 Stockholm.
3 These figures are drawn from two 2001 Census tables published on-line by Statistics Canada. See the tables "Labour Force Activity (8), Presence of Children by Age Groups (11), Age Groups (5A), Marital Status (7C) and Sex (3) for Population 15 Years and Over Living in Private Households, for Canada, Provinces, Territories, Census Metropolitan Areas and Census Agglomerations, 2001 Census – 20% Sample Data" and "Hours Spent Providing Unpaid Care or Assistance to Seniors (7), Selected Labour Force, Demographic, Cultural, Educational and Income Characteristics (312) and Sex (3) for Population 15 Years and Over, for Canada, Provinces, Territories, Census Metropolitan Areas and Census Agglomerations, 1996 and 2001 Censuses – 20% Sample Data." The first table can be found at http://www12.statcan.ca/english/census01/products/standard/themes/ (Table 28,

under "Canada's Workforce: Paid Work"). The second table is available at http://www12.statcan.ca/english/census01/products/standard/themes/ (Table 13, under "Canada's Workforce: Unpaid Work").

4 This author calculation is based on figures from Tables 93f0027xdb96006v2.ivt and 93f0027xdb96016v2.ivt of the 1996 Census, Nation Series, Package 7 – "Labour Market Activities ... Household Activities, Place of Work, Mode of Transportation." See http://data.library.ubc.ca/datalib/survey/statscan/census/1996/b2020/nation/index.html#pack7.

5 Baril, Lefebvre, and Merrigan's (2000, 5) limited attention to the systemic factors that influence the patriarchal division of labour is conspicuous in its absence from their discussion of reasons for governments to deliver public subsidies to "people who have made the private choice to have children." Their analysis references such positions as how "society ... needs children" since they "are the source of renewal of the human capital of an economy"; how "equal opportunity" for children requires the redistribution of material rewards from rich to poor families; as well as the difficulties that parents encounter balancing work and family. However, the discussion makes no reference to the gender division of labour or the barriers to gender, race, and class equality that this division poses.

Chapter 8: The Politics of Time

1 Some material in Chapters 7 and 8 has been revised from an earlier version that appeared in "The Politics of Time: Integrating a Richer Appreciation for Work Family Balance into the Canadian Welfare Regime," *Canadian Review of Social Policy* 49-50: 113-38. The author is grateful for the journal's permission to revise the passages for this book.

References

Adriaansens, Hans. 1994. "Citizenship, Work and Welfare." In *The Condition of Citizenship*, edited by B.V. Steenbergen. London: Sage.

Advisory Group. 1994. "Report of the Advisory Group on Working Time and the Distribution of Work." Ottawa: Human Resources Development Canada/ Ministry of Supply and Services Canada.

Arat-Koc, Sedef. 1997. "From 'Mothers of the Nation' to Migrant Workers." In *Not One of the Family: Foreign Domestic Workers in Canada*, edited by A.B. Bakan and D. Stasiulis. Toronto: University of Toronto Press.

Armstrong, Pat. 1997. "Restructuring Public and Private: Women's Paid and Unpaid Work." In *Challenging the Public/Private Divide: Feminism, Law, and Public Policy*, edited by S. Boyd. Toronto: University of Toronto Press.

Baier, Annette. 1985. *Postures of the Mind: Essays on Mind and Morals*. Minneapolis: University of Minnesota Press.

Bakan, Abigail B., and Daiva Stasiulis. 1997a. "Introduction." In *Not One of the Family: Foreign Domestic Workers in Canada*, edited by A.B. Bakan and D. Stasiulis. Toronto: University of Toronto Press.

–. 1997b. "Foreign Domestic Worker Policy in Canada and the Social Boundaries of Modern Citizenship." In *Not One of the Family: Foreign Domestic Workers in Canada*, edited by A.B. Bakan and D. Stasiulis. Toronto: University of Toronto Press.

Bakan, Joel. 1997. *Just Words: Constitutional Rights and Social Wrongs*. Toronto: University of Toronto Press.

Baker, Maureen. 1995. *Canadian Family Policies: Cross-National Comparisons*. Toronto: University of Toronto Press.

–. 1997. "Parental Benefit Policies and the Gendered Division of Labor." *Social Service Review* 71 (1): 51-71.

Bakker, Isabella, ed. 1996. *Rethinking Restructuring: Gender and Change in Canada*. Toronto: University of Toronto Press.

Banting, Keith. 1982. *The Welfare State and Canadian Federalism*. Montreal and Kingston: McGill-Queen's University Press.

Barbalet, J.M. 1988. *Citizenship: Rights, Struggle, and Class Inequality*. Milton Keynes, UK: Open University Press.

Barclay, Lesley, and Deborah Lupton. 1999. "The Experiences of New Fatherhood: A Socio-Cultural Analysis." *Journal of Advanced Nursing* 29 (4): 1013-20.

Baril, Robert, Pierre Lefebvre, and Philip Merrigan. 2000. "Quebec Family Policy: Impact and Options." *Choices* 6 (1): 1-52.

Baum, Charles. 2002. "A Dynamic Analysis of the Effect of Child Care Costs on the Work Decisions of Low-Income Mothers with Infants." *Demography* 39 (1): 139-64.

Beaudry, Paul, and David Green. 2000. "Cohort Patterns in Canadian Earnings: Assessing the Role of Skill Premia in Inequality Trends." *Canadian Journal of Economics* 33 (4): 907-36.

Beaujot, Rod. 2000. *Earning and Caring in Canadian Families*. Peterborough, ON: Broadview Press.

Becker, Gary. 1981. *A Treatise on the Family*. Cambridge, MA: Harvard University Press.

Berger, Brigitte, and Peter L. Berger. 1983. *The War over the Family: Capturing the Middle Ground*. Garden City, NY: Anchor Press/Doubleday.

Bergman, Helena, and Barbara Hobson. 2002. "Compulsory Fatherhood: The Coding of Fatherhood in the Swedish Welfare State." In *Making Men into Fathers: Men, Masculinities and the Social Politics of Fatherhood*, edited by B. Hobson. Cambridge: Cambridge University Press.

Berrueta-Clement, John, Lawrence Schweinhart, W. Steven Barnett, Ann Epstein, and David Weikart. 1984. *Changed Lives: The Effects of the Perry Preschool Program on Youths through Age 19*. Ypsilanti, MI: High/Scope Educational Research Foundation.

Bilous, Alexandre. 2000. *Law on the 35-Hour Week Is in Force* (ID: FR0001137F). European Industrial Relations Observatory Online. Available from http://www.eiro.eurofound.ie/2000/01/feature/FR0001137F.html.

Bluestone, Barry, and Stephen Rose. 2000. "The Enigma of Working Time Trends." In *Working Time: International Trends, Theory and Policy Perspectives*, edited by L. Golden and D.M. Figart. New York: Routledge.

Boris, Eileen. 1994. "Mothers Are Not Workers: Homework Regulation and the Construction of Motherhood, 1948-1953." In *Mothering: Ideology, Experience, and Agency*, edited by E.N. Glenn, G. Chang, and L.R. Forcey. New York: Routledge.

Bosch, Gerhard. 1993. "Federal Republic of Germany." In *Times Are Changing: Working Time in 14 Industrialized Countries*, edited by G. Bosch, P. Dawkins, and F. Michon. Geneva: International Institute for Labour Studies.

Bourdieu, Pierre. 1980. "Le Capital Social." *Actes de la Recherche en Sciences Sociales* 31.

Bradshaw, Jonathan, and Naomi Finch. 2002. "A Comparison of Child Benefit Packages in 22 Countries." Leeds: UK Department for Work and Pensions.

Brandth, Berit, and Elin Kvande. 1998. "Masculinity and Child Care: The Reconstruction of Fathering." *Sociological Review* 46 (2): 293-313.

Brisson C., N. Laflamme, J. Moisan, A. Milot, B. Mâsse, and M. Vézina. 1999. "Effect of Family Responsibilities and Job Strain on Ambulatory Blood Pressure among White-Collar Women." *Psychosomatic Medicine* 61 (2): 205-13.

Broberg, Anders G., Holger Wessels, Michael E. Lamb, and C. Philip Hwang. 1997. "Effects of Day Care on the Development of Cognitive Abilities in 8-Year-Olds: A Longitudinal Study." *Developmental Psychology* 33 (1): 62-69.

Brodie, Janine. 1995. *Politics on the Margins: Restructuring and the Canadian Women's Movement*. Halifax: Fernwood Press.

–. 1996. "Restructuring and the New Citizenship." In *Rethinking Restructuring: Gender and Change in Canada,* edited by I. Bakker. Toronto: University of Toronto Press.

–. 1997. "Meso-Discourses, State Forms and the Gendering of Liberal-Democratic Citizenship." *Citizenship Studies* 1 (2): 223-42.

Bussemaker, Jet. 1998. "Vocabularies of Citizenship and Gender: The Netherlands." *Critical Social Policy* 18 (3): 333-54.

Bussemaker, Jet, and Rian Voet. 1998. "Citizenship and Gender: Theoretical Approaches and Historical Legacies." *Critical Social Policy* 18 (3): 277-308.

Canada Employment Insurance Commission. 2003. "Employment Insurance: 2002 Monitoring and Assessment Report." Hull, QC: Human Resources Development Canada, Strategic Policy, Labour Market Policy Directorate.

Card, Claudia. 1988. "Women's Values and Ethical Ideals: Must We Mean What We Say?" *Ethics* 99: 125-35.

Cass, Bettina. 1994. "Citizenship, Work and Welfare: The Dilemma of Australian Women." *Social Politics* 1 (1): 106-24.

Chief Actuary. 2001. "Report on Employment Insurance." Ottawa: Human Resources Development Canada.

Childcare Resource and Research Unit (CRRU). 2000. *Early Childhood Care and Education in Canada: Provinces and Territories 1998.* Toronto: Child Resource and Research Unit, Centre for Urban and Community Studies, University of Toronto.

Cleveland, Gordon, Morley Gunderson, and Douglas Hyatt. 1996. "Child Care Costs and the Employment Decisions of Women: Canadian Evidence." *Canadian Journal of Economics* 29 (1): 132-51.

Cleveland, Gordon, and Douglas Hyatt. 2002. "Child Care Workers' Wages: New Evidence on Returns to Education, Experience, Job Tenure and Auspice." *Journal of Population Economics* 15 (3): 575-97.

Cleveland, Gordon, and Michael Krashinsky. 1998. *The Benefits and Costs of Good Child Care: The Economic Rationale for Public Investment in Young Children.* Toronto: Childcare Resource and Research Unit, Centre for Urban and Community Studies, University of Toronto.

Code, Lorraine. 1987. "Second Persons." *Canadian Journal of Philosophy* 13 (Supplementary): 357-82.

Collins, Patricia Hill. 1991. *Black Feminist Thought: Knowledge, Consciousness, and the Politics of Empowerment.* New York/London: Routledge Press.

–. 1994. "Shifting the Center: Race, Class, and Feminist Theorizing about Motherhood." In *Mothering: Ideology, Experience, and Agency,* edited by E.N. Glenn, G. Chang, and L.R. Forcey. New York: Routledge.

Coltrane, Scott. 1996. *Family Man: Fatherhood, Housework and Gender Equity.* New York: Oxford University Press.

Connell, R.W. 1995. *Masculinities.* Cambridge UK: Polity Press.

Contensou, François, and Radu Vranceanu. 2000. *Working Time: Theory and Policy Implications.* Northampton, MA: Edward Elgar Publishing.

Conway, John F. 1997. *The Canadian Family in Crisis.* 3rd ed. Toronto: James Lorimer and Company.

Courchene, Thomas J. 1994a. *Social Canada in the Millennium: Reform Imperatives and Restructuring Principles.* Toronto: C.D. Howe Institute/Renouf Publishing Company.

–. 1994b. "Canada's Social Policy Deficit: Implications for Fiscal Federalism." In *The Future of Fiscal Federalism*, edited by K.G. Banting, D.M. Brown, and T.J. Courchene. Kingston, ON: Queen's University School of Policy Studies.

–. 1997. "ACCESS: A Convention on the Canadian Economic and Social Systems." In *Assessing ACCESS: Towards a New Social Union*. Kingston, ON: Institute of Intergovernmental Relations, Queen's University.

–. 2001. *A State of Minds: Toward a Human Capital Future for Canadians*. Montreal: Institute for Research on Public Policy.

Cox, Robert Henry. 1998. "From Safety Net to Trampoline: Labor Market Activation in the Netherlands and Denmark." *Governance: An International Journal of Policy and Administration* 11 (4): 397-414.

Coyne, Andrew. 1999. "Taxes – A Motherhood Issue." *National Post*, 10 March, A19.

Daly, Mary, and Jane Lewis. 1998. "Introduction: Conceptualising Social Care in the Context of Welfare State Restructuring." In *Gender, Social Care and Welfare State Restructuring in Europe*, edited by J. Lewis. Aldershot, UK: Ashgate Publishing.

Denton, Frank T., and Byron G. Spencer. 1999. "Population Aging and Its Economic Costs: A Survey of the Issues and Evidence." QSEP Research Report No. 340. Hamilton, ON: Research Institute for Quantitative Studies in Economics and Population, Faculty of Social Sciences, McMaster University.

Dillon, Robin. 1992. "Care and Respect." In *Explorations in Feminist Ethics: Theory and Practice*, edited by E. Browning Cole and S. Coultrap-McQuin. Bloomington, IN: Indiana University Press.

Drolet, Marie. 2002a. "New Evidence on Gender Pay Differentials: Does Measurement Matter?" *Canadian Public Policy* 28 (1): 1-16.

–. 2002b. "Wives, Mothers and Wages: Does Timing Matter?" Ottawa: Statistics Canada, Business and Labour Market Analysis Division. Catalogue no. 11F0019M1E – No. 186.

Drolet, Marie, and René Morissette. 1997. "Working More? Less? What Do Workers Prefer?" *Perspectives on Labour and Income* (winter): 32-38.

Dua, Enakshi. 1999. "Beyond Diversity: Exploring the Ways in Which the Discourse of Race Has Shaped the Institution of the Nuclear Family." In *Scratching the Surface: Canadian Anti-Racist Feminist Thought*, edited by E. Dua and A. Robertson. Toronto: Women's Press.

Duchesne, Doreen. 1997. "Working Overtime in Today's Labour Market." *Perspectives on Labour and Income* (winter): 9-24.

Duxbury, Linda, and Chris Higgins. 2003. "Where to Work in Canada? An Examination of Regional Differences in Work-Life Practices." Vancouver: BC Council of the Families.

Dwyer, Peter. 2000. *Welfare Rights and Responsibilities*. Bristol, UK: Policy Press.

Eggebeen, David J., and Chris Knoester. 2001. "Does Fatherhood Matter for Men?" *Journal of Marriage and Family* 63 (May): 381-93.

Eichler, Margrit. 1997. *Family Shifts: Families, Policies and Gender Equality*. Don Mills, ON: Oxford University Press.

Elshtain, Jean Bethke. 1981. *Public Man, Private Woman: Women in Social and Political Thought*. Princeton, NJ: Princeton University Press.

Esping-Andersen, Gøsta. 1990. *The Three Worlds of Welfare Capitalism*. Cambridge, UK: Polity Press.

–. 1999. *Social Foundations of Postindustrial Economies*. Oxford, UK: Oxford University Press.

–. 2002. *Why We Need a New Welfare State*. Oxford, UK: Oxford University Press.

Etzioni, Amitai. 1993. *The Spirit of Community*. New York: Crown Publishers.

–. 1996. *The New Golden Rule: Community and Morality in a Democratic Society*. New York: Basic Books.

European Industrial Relations Review. 1998. "Making Way for the 35-Hour Working Week. *European Industrial Relations Review (EIRR)* 294 (July): 19-25.

–. 2001a. "Maternity, Paternity and Parental Benefits across Europe – Part 2." *EIRR* 330 (July): 15-18.

–. 2001b. "Maternity, Paternity and Parental Benefits across Europe – Part 3." *EIRR* 331 (August): 13-17.

–. 2001c. "New 35-Hour Week for Small Companies." *EIRR* 335 (December): 26-28.

Evans, Patricia M., and Gerda R. Wekerle, eds. 1997. *Women and the Canadian Welfare State: Challenges and Change*. Toronto: University of Toronto Press.

Evers, Adelbert, Marja Pilj, and Clare Ungerson, eds. 1994. *Payments for Care: A Comparative Overview*. Aldershot, UK: Avebury.

Forer, Barry, and Theresa Hunter. 2001. "2001 Provincial Child Care Survey: Final Report." Victoria: Ministry of Community, Aboriginal and Women's Services, Child Care Policy Branch.

Fraser, Nancy. 1994. "After the Family Wage: Gender Equity and the Welfare State." *Political Theory* 22 (4): 591-618.

–. 1997. *Justice Interruptus: Critical Reflections on the "Postsocialist" Condition*. New York: Routledge.

Freeman, Richard B. 1998. "Work-Sharing to Full Employment: Serious Option or Populist Fallacy?" In *Generating Jobs: How to Increase Demand for Less-Skilled Workers*, edited by R.B. Freeman and P. Gottschalk. New York: Russell Sage Foundation.

Friedan, Betty. 1963. *The Feminine Mystique*. New York: Norton.

Friedman, Marilyn. 1993. "Beyond Caring: The De-Moralization of Gender." In *An Ethic of Care*, edited by M.J. Larrabee. New York: Routledge.

Friendly, Martha, Jane Beach, and Michelle Turiano. 2002. *Early Childhood Education and Care in Canada 2001*. Toronto: Childcare Resource and Research Unit, University of Toronto.

Fudge, Judy. 1997. "Little Victories and Big Defeats: The Rise and Fall of Collective Bargaining Rights for Domestic Workers in Ontario." In *Not One of the Family: Foreign Domestic Workers in Canada*, edited by A.B. Bakan and D. Stasiulis. Toronto: University of Toronto Press.

Gagné, Linda. 2003. *Parental Work, Child-Care Use and Young Children's Cognitive Outcomes*. Statistics Canada. Available from http://www.statcan.ca/english/research/89-594-XIE/89-594-XIE.pdf.

Gairdner, William D. 1992. *The War against the Family*. Toronto: Stoddart Publishing.

Gaskell, Jane. 1991. "What Counts as Skill? Reflections on Pay Equity." In *Just Wages: A Feminist Assessment of Pay Equity*, edited by J. Fudge and P. McDermott. Toronto: University of Toronto Press.

Giddens, Anthony. 1994. *Beyond Left and Right: The Future of Radical Politics*. Stanford, CA: Stanford University Press.

–. 1999. *The Third Way*. Cambridge, UK: Polity Press.

–. 2000. *The Third Way and Its Critics*. Cambridge, UK: Polity Press.

Gilder, George. 1986. *Men and Marriage*. London: Buchan and Enright.

–. 1987. "Welfare's 'New Consensus': The Collapse of the American Family." *The Public Interest* (89): 20-25.

Gilligan, Carol. 1982. *In a Different Voice: Psychological Theory and Women's Development*. Cambridge, MA: Harvard University Press.

–. 1987. "Moral Orientation and Moral Development." In *Women and Moral Theory*, edited by E.F. Kittay and D.T. Meyers. Totowa, NJ: Rowman and Littlefield.

–. 1995. "Hearing the Difference: Theorizing Connection." *Hypatia* 10: 120-27.

Glenn, Evelyn Nakano. 1994. "Social Constructions of Mothering: A Thematic Overview." In *Mothering: Ideology, Experience, and Agency*, edited by E.N. Glenn, G. Chang, and L.R. Forcey. New York: Routledge.

Government of British Columbia. 2002. "Ministry of Human Resources Service Plan Summary: 2002/03-2004/05." Victoria: Ministry of Human Resources.

Government of Canada. 2000. *Economic Statement and Budget Update*. Ottawa: Department of Finance. Available from http://www.fin.gc.ca/ec2000/ectoce.htm.

–. 2004. *Canada Pension Plan/Old Age Security Statistical Bulletin October 2004*. Ottawa: Social Development Canada. Available from http://www.hrsdc.gc.ca/en/isp/statistics/pdf/statbulletin1004.pdf.

Government of Ontario. 2000. *Employment Standards Reform: Hours of Work*. Toronto: Ministry of Labour. Available from http://www.gov.on.ca/lab/ann/00-48be.htm.

Government of Quebec. 2001. "Rapport Annuel 2000-2001." Quebec, QC: Ministère de la Famille et de l'enfance.

Government of Saskatchewan. 2002. *Benefits for Part-Time Employees*. Regina: Saskatchewan Ministry of Labour. Available from www.labour.gov.sk.ca/standards/guide/benefits.htm.

Gramsci, Antonio. 1971. *Selections from the Prison Notebooks*. Edited by Q. Hoare and G.N. Smith. New York: International Publishers.

Gray, John. 2000. "Inclusion: A Radical Critique." In *Social Inclusion: Possibilities and Tensions*, edited by P. Askonas and A. Stewart. London: Macmillan.

Hale, Geoffrey E. 2002. *The Politics of Taxation in Canada*. Peterborough, ON: Broadview Press.

Hall, Karen. 1999. "Hours Polarization at the End of the 1990s." *Perspectives on Labour and Income* 11, 2 (summer): 28-37.

Hayden, Anders. 1999. *Sharing the Work, Sparing the Planet: Work Time, Consumption, and Ecology*. Toronto: Between the Lines.

Heckman, James, and Lance Lochner. 2000. "Rethinking Education and Training Policy." In *Securing the Future: Investing in Children from Birth to College*, edited by S. Danziger and J. Waldfogel. New York: Russell Sage.

Held, Virginia. 1995. "The Meshing of Care and Justice." *Hypatia* 10: 128-32.

Hertzman, Clyde. 2002. "Leave No Child Behind: Social Exclusion and Child Development." Toronto: Laidlaw Foundation.

Hirschl, Ran. 2000. "'Negative' Rights vs. 'Positive' Entitlements: A Comparative Study of Judicial Interpretations of Rights in an Emerging Neo-Liberal Economic Order." *Human Rights Quarterly* 22: 1060-98.

Hobson, Barbara, ed. 2002. *Making Men into Fathers: Men, Masculinities and the Social Politics of Fatherhood*. Cambridge, UK: Cambridge University Press.

Højgaard, Lis. 1997. "Working Fathers – Caught in the Web of the Symbolic Order of Gender." *Acta Sociologica* 40: 245-62.

Huberman, Michael, and Paul Lanoie. 2000. "Changing Attitudes toward Worksharing." *Canadian Public Policy* 26 (2): 141-56.

Hunt, Alan. 1993. *Explorations in Law and Society: Towards a Constitutive Theory of Law*. New York: Routledge.

Hunt, Jennifer. 1998. "Hours Reductions as Work-Sharing." *Brookings Papers on Economic Activity* 1: 339-81.

–. 1999. "Has Work-Sharing Worked in Germany?" *Quarterly Journal of Economics* 114 (1): 117-48.

Iyer, Nitya. 1997. "Some Mothers Are Better than Others: A Re-Examination of Maternity Benefits." In *Challenging the Public/Private Divide: Feminism, Law, and Public Policy*, edited by S. Boyd. Toronto: University of Toronto Press.

Jackman, Martha. 2000. "What's Wrong with Social and Economic Rights?" *Constitutional Law* 11 (2): 235-46.

Jacobs, E.V., G. Selig, and D.R. White. 1992. "Classroom Behaviour in Grade One: Does the Quality of Preschool Day Care Experience Make a Difference?" *Canadian Journal of Research in Early Childhood Education* 3: 89-100.

Jacobs, Jerry A., and Kathleen Gerson. 2000. "Who Are the Overworked Americans?" In *Working Time: International Trends, Theory and Policy Perspectives*, edited by L. Golden and D.M. Figart. New York: Routledge.

Jenson, Jane. 1997a. "Fated to Live in Interesting Times: Canada's Changing Citizenship Regimes." *Canadian Journal of Political Science* 30 (4): 627-44.

–. 1997b. "Who Cares? Gender and Welfare Regimes." *Social Politics* 4 (2): 182-87.

–. 2003. "Converging, Diverging or Shifting? Social Architecture in an Era of Change." Paper read at Canadian Political Science Association Annual Meetings, May 2003, Halifax, NS.

Jenson, Jane, and Susan D. Phillips. 1996. "Regime Shift: New Citizenship Practices in Canada." *International Journal of Canadian Studies* 14 (Fall): 111-35.

Jenson, Jane, and Denis Saint-Martin. 2003. "New Routes to Social Cohesion? Citizenship and the Social Investment State." *Canadian Journal of Sociology* 28 (1): 77-99.

Jenson, Jane, and Mariette Sineau. 2001. *Who Cares? Women's Work, Childcare and Welfare State Redesign*. Toronto: University of Toronto Press.

Kamo, Yoshinori, and Ellen L. Cohen. 1998. "Division of Household Work between Partners: A Comparison of Black and White Couples." *Journal of Comparative Family Studies* 29 (1): 131-45.

Kant, Immanuel. 1993. *Grounding for the Metaphysics of Morals*. Translated by J.W. Ellington. Indianapolis IN: Hackett Publishing. Original edition published in 1785.

Kershaw, Paul. 2002. "Beyond the Spousal Tax Credit: Rethinking the Tax Treatment of Caregiving and Dependency (Again!) in the Light of the Law Commission Report." *Canadian Tax Journal* 50 (6): 1949-78.

–. 2004. "'Choice' Discourse in BC Child Care: Distancing Policy from Research." *Canadian Journal of Political Science* 37 (4): 927-50.

Kimmel, Jean. 1998. "Child Care Costs as a Barrier to Employment for Single and Married Mothers." *Review of Economics and Statistics* 80 (2): 287-99.

King, Desmond S., and Jeremy Waldron. 1988. "Citizenship, Social Citizenship and the Defence of Welfare Provision." *British Journal of Political Science* 18: 415-43.

Klein, Seth, and Andrea Long. 2003. "A Bad Time to Be Poor." Vancouver: Canadian Centre for Policy Alternatives/Social Planning and Research Council of BC.

Kline, Marlee. 1995. "Complicating the Ideology of Motherhood: Child Welfare Law and First Nation Women." In *Mothers in Law: Feminist Theory and the Legal Regulation of Motherhood,* edited by M.A. Fineman and I. Karpin. New York: Columbia University Press.

–. 1997. "Blue Meanies in Alberta: Tory Tactics and the Privatization of Child Welfare." In *Challenging the Public/Private Divide: Feminism, Law, and Public Policy,* edited by S. Boyd. Toronto: University of Toronto Press.

Knijn, Trudie. 1994. "Fish without Bikes: Revision of the Dutch Welfare State and Its Consequences for the (In)dependence of Single Mothers." *Social Politics* 1 (1): 83-105.

Knijn, Trudie, and Monique Kremer. 1997. "Gender and the Caring Dimension of Welfare States: Toward Inclusive Citizenship." *Social Politics* 4 (3): 328-61.

Knijn, Trudie, and Peter Selten. 2002. "Transformations of Fatherhood: The Netherlands." In *Making Men into Fathers: Men, Masculinities and the Social Politics of Fatherhood,* edited by B. Hobson. Cambridge: Cambridge University Press.

Kymlicka, Will. 1989. *Liberalism, Community and Culture.* Oxford, UK: Clarendon Press.

–. 2002. *Contemporary Political Philosophy: An Introduction.* 2nd ed. Oxford, UK: Oxford University Press.

Kymlicka, Will, and Wayne Norman. 1994. "Return of the Citizen: A Survey of Recent Work on Citizenship Theory." *Ethics* 104 (January): 352-81.

–. 2000. "Citizenship in Culturally Diverse Societies: Issues, Contexts, Concepts." In *Citizenship in Diverse Societies,* edited by W. Kymlicka and W. Norman. Oxford, UK: Oxford University Press.

–. 2003. "Citizenship." In *A Companion to Applied Ethics,* edited by R.G. Frey and C.H. Wellman. Oxford, UK: Blackwell Publishing.

Langan, Mary, and Ilona Ostner. 1991. "Gender and Welfare." In *Towards a European Welfare State?* edited by G. Room. Bristol, UK: SAUS Publications.

Lanoie, Paul, and F. Raymond. 1999. "Subvention gouvernementale et partagae du travail: une analyse économique – Part 2." Montreal: Centre for Inter-university Research and Analysis on Organizations.

Larner, Wendy. 2000. "Post-Welfare State Governance: Towards a Code of Social and Family Responsibility." *Social Politics* 7 (2): 244-65.

Laycock, David. 2002. *The New Right and Democracy in Canada: Understanding Reform and the Canadian Alliance.* Don Mills, ON: Oxford University Press.

Leblanc, Daniel. 1999. "Nanny Faces Deportation for Doing Too Many Jobs." *Globe and Mail,* 20 July, A1-A2.

Leira, Arnlaug. 1998. "Caring as Social Right: Cash for Child Care and Daddy Leave." *Social Politics* 5 (3): 362-78.

Levitas, Ruth. 1998. *The Inclusive Society? Social Exclusion and New Labour.* London: Macmillan.

Lewis, Jane. 2001. "The Decline of the Male Breadwinner Model: Implications for Work and Care." *Social Politics* 8 (2): 152-69.

Lister, Ruth. 1997a. *Citizenship: Feminist Perspectives.* London: Macmillan.

–. 1997b. "Dialectics of Citizenship." *Hypatia* 12 (4): 6-26.

–. 1998. "Vocabularies of Citizenship and Gender: The UK." *Critical Social Policy* 18 (3): 309-31.

–. 2000a. "Dilemmas in Engendering Citizenship." In *Gender and Citizenship in Transition,* edited by B. Hobson. London: Macmillan.

–. 2000b. "Strategies for Social Inclusion: Promoting Social Cohesion or Social Justice?" In *Social Inclusion: Possibilities and Tensions,* edited by P. Askonas and A. Stewart. London: Macmillan.

Lupton, Deborah, and Lesley Barclay. 1997. *Constructing Fatherhood: Discourses and Experiences.* London: Sage.

Luxton, Meg, and Ester Reiter. 1997. "Double, Double, Toil and Trouble ... Women's Experience of Work and Family in Canada 1980-1995." In *Women and the Canadian Welfare State: Challenges and Change,* edited by P.M. Evans and G.R. Wekerle. Toronto: University of Toronto Press.

MacIntyre, Alasdair. 1984. *After Virtue.* 2nd ed. Notre Dame, IN: University of Notre Dame Press.

McBride, Stephen, and John Shields. 1997. *Dismantling a Nation: The Transition to Corporate Rule in Canada.* 2nd ed. Halifax: Fernwood Press.

McCarthy, Shawn. 1999a. "Reform Party Calls for Tax Breaks for Parents Staying Home with Children." *Globe and Mail,* 5 March, A2.

–. 1999b. "MPs to Vote on Reform Party Tax Motion." *Globe and Mail,* March 8, A4.

Maloney, Maureen A. 1989. "Women and the Income Tax Act: Marriage, Motherhood, and Divorce." *Canadian Journal of Women and the Law* 3: 182-210.

Mann, Michael. 1987. "Ruling Class Strategies and Citizenship." *Sociology* 21 (3): 339-54.

Marshall, Katherine. 2003. "Benefiting from Extended Parental Leave." *Perspectives on Labour and Income* (March): 5-11.

Marshall, T.H. 1964. *Class, Citizenship, and Social Development.* Garden City, NY: Doubleday.

–. 1981. *The Right to Welfare and Other Essays.* New York: Free Press/Macmillan.

Martin, Claude. 1996. "French Review Article: The Debate in France over 'Social Exclusion.'" *Social Policy and Administration* 30 (4): 382-92.

Mason, Melodie. 1999. "Ontario Works and Single Mothers: Redefining 'Deservedness and the Social Contract.'" *Journal of Canadian Studies* 34 (2): 89-102.

Masse, Leonard M., and Steven Barnett. 2002. *A Benefit Cost Analysis of the Abecedarian Early Childhood Intervention.* New Brunswick, NJ: National Institute for Early Education Research. Available from http://nieer.org/resources/research/AbecedarianStudy.pdf.

Mazankowski, Don. 2001. "A Framework for Reform: Report of the Premier's Advisory Council on Health." Edmonton: Government of Alberta.

Mead, Lawrence M. 1986. *Beyond Entitlement: The Social Obligations of Citizenship.* New York: Free Press/Macmillan.

–. 1997a. "Citizenship and Social Policy: T.H. Marshall and Poverty." *Social Philosophy and Policy* 14 (2): 197-230.

–, ed. 1997b. *The New Paternalism*. Washington, DC: Brookings Institute Press.

Mill, John Stuart. 1975. *On Liberty*. Edited by D. Spitz. New York: Norton.

Mink, Gwendolyn. 2002. *Welfare's End*. Revised ed. Ithaca, NY: Cornell University Press.

Misra, Joya, and Frances Akins. 1998. "The Welfare State and Women: Structure, Agency, and Diversity." *Social Politics* 5 (3): 259-85.

Mitchell, Alanna, and Brian Laghi. 2000. "Filipina Nanny Agrees to Leave Canada: Apparent Compromise Means She Will Receive Special Ministerial Permission to Return." *Globe and Mail,* February 17, A2.

Morissette, René, John Myles, and Garnett Picot. 1995. "Earnings Polarization in Canada, 1969-1991." In *Labour Market Polarization and Social Policy Reform,* edited by K.G. Banting and C.M. Beach. Kingston, ON: Queen's University School of Policy Studies.

Moss, Peter, and Helen Penn. 1996. *Transforming Nursery Education*. London: Paul Chapman Publishing.

Murray, Charles. 1984. *Losing Ground: American Social Policy, 1950-1980*. New York: Basic Books.

–. 1987. "In Search of the Working Poor." *Public Interest* 89 (fall): 3-19.

Mutari, Ellen, and Deborah M. Figart. 2001. "Europe at a Crossroads: Harmonization, Liberalization, and the Gender of Work Time." *Social Politics* 8 (1): 36-64.

Narayan, Uma. 1995. "Colonialism and Its Others: Considerations on Rights and Care Discourses." *Hypatia* 10: 133-40.

National Council of Welfare. 2000. *Poverty Profile 1998*. Ottawa: Minister of Public Works and Government Services. Available from http://www.ncwcnbes.net/htmdocument/reportpovertypro98/poverty98_e.htm.

–. 2002. *Poverty Profile 1999*. Ottawa: National Council of Welfare. Available from http://www.ncwcnbes.net/htmdocument/reportpovertypro99/Introduction_e.htm.

Norrie McCain, Margaret, and Fraser Mustard. 1999. "Early Years Study: Reversing the Real Brain Drain." Toronto: Canadian Institute for Advanced Research.

O'Connor, Julia S. 1993. "Gender, Class and Citizenship in the Comparative Analysis of Welfare State Regimes: Theoretical and Methodological Issues." *British Journal of Sociology* 44, 3 (September): 501-18.

O'Connor, Julia S., Ann Shola Orloff, and Sheila Shaver. 1999. *States, Markets, Families: Gender, Liberalism and Social Policy in Australia, Canada, Great Britain and the United States*. Cambridge: Cambridge University Press.

O'Hara, Kathy. 1998. *Comparative Family Policies: Eight Countries' Stories*. Ottawa: Canadian Policy Research Network.

Okin, Susan Moller. 1989. *Justice, Gender and the Family*. New York: Basic Books.

Oldfield, Adrian. 1990. *Citizenship and Community: Civic Republicanism and the Modern World*. London: Routledge.

–. 1998. "Citizenship and Community: Civic Republicanism and the Modern World." In *The Citizenship Debates*, edited by G. Shafir. Minneapolis: University of Minnesota Press.

Olson, Kevin. 2002. "Recognizing Gender, Redistributing Labor." *Social Politics* 9 (3): 380-410.

Organisation for Economic Co-operation and Development. 1999. *A Caring World: The New Social Policy Agenda*. Paris: OECD.

Orloff, Ann Shola. 1993. "Gender and the Social Rights of Citizenship: The Comparative Analysis of Gender Relations and Welfare States." *American Sociological Review* 58 (June): 303-28.

–. 1997. "Comment on Jane Lewis's 'Gender and Welfare Regimes: Further Thoughts.'" *Social Politics* 4 (2): 188-202.

Orloff, Ann Shola, and Renee A. Monson. 2002. "Citizens, Workers or Fathers? Men in the History of US Social Policy." In *Making Men into Fathers: Men, Masculinities and the Social Politics of Fatherhood,* edited by B. Hobson. Cambridge: Cambridge University Press.

Osberg, Lars. 2001. "Labour Supply and Inequality Trends in the USA and Elsewhere." Paper read at CSLS/IRPP Conference on Linkages between Economic Growth and Inequality, 26 January 2001, at Château Laurier Hotel, Ottawa.

Parry, Geraint, George Moyser, and Neil Day. 1992. *Political Participation and Democracy in Britain.* Cambridge: Cambridge University Press.

Pateman, Carole. 1988. *The Sexual Contract.* Cambridge, UK: Polity Press.

–. 1989. *The Disorder of Women.* Stanford, CA: Stanford University Press.

Peisner-Feinberg, E.S., M.R. Burchinal, R.M. Clifford, M.L. Culkin, C. Howes, and S.L. Kagan. 1999. "The Children of the Cost, Quality and Outcomes Study Go to School. Executive Summary." Chapel Hill: Frank Porter Graham Child Development Center, University of North Carolina.

Pérusse, Dominique. 2003. "New Maternity and Parental Benefits." *Perspectives on Labour and Income* (March): 12-15.

Phillips, Paul, and Erin Phillips. 1993. *Women and Work: Inequality in the Canadian Labour Market.* Toronto: James Lorimer and Company.

Picot, G. 1998. "What Is Happening to Earnings Inequality and Youth Wages in the 1990s?" *Canadian Economic Observer* (September): 3.1-3.18.

Pierson, Paul. 2001. "Investigating the Welfare State at Century's End." In *The New Politics of the Welfare State,* edited by P. Pierson. Oxford, UK: Oxford University Press.

Popenoe, David. 1996. *Life without Father.* New York: Free Press.

Powell, Lisa. 1997. "Family Behaviour and Child Care Costs: Policy Implications." *Policy Options* 18 (1): 11-15.

Putnam, Robert. 2000. *Bowling Alone: The Collapse and Revival of American Community.* New York: Simon and Schuster.

Ratcliffe, Peter. 2000. "Is the Assertion of Minority Identity Compatible with the Idea of a Socially Inclusive Society?" In *Social Inclusion: Possibilities and Tensions,* edited by P. Askonas and A. Stewart. London: Macmillan.

Rawls, John. 1971. *A Theory of Justice.* Cambridge, MA: Harvard University Press.

–. 1993. *Political Liberalism.* New York: Columbia University Press.

REAL Women of Canada. 1999. "Giving Birth and Returning to Paid Employment." *REALity* 18 (5). Available from http://www.realwomenca.com/newsletter/1999_Sept_Oct/article_3.html.

–. 2001. *Statement on Child Care.* Available from http://www.realwomenca.com/papers/child_care.htm.

Rees, Anthony M. 1995. "The Promise of Social Citizenship." *Policy and Politics* 23 (4): 313-25.

Ribar, David C. 1995. "A Structural Model of Child Care and the Labor Supply of Married Women." *Journal of Labor Economics* 13 (3): 558-97.

Richards, John. 1994. "The Case for Cutting the Public Sector Payroll." In *The Future of Fiscal Federalism*, edited by K.G. Banting, D.M. Brown, and T.J. Courchene. Kingston, ON: Queen's University School of Policy Studies.

–. 1997. *Retooling the Welfare State: What's Right, What's Wrong, What's to Be Done*. Toronto: C.D. Howe Institute/Renouf Publishing Company.

Roberts, Dorothy E. 1995a. "Racism and Patriarchy in the Meaning of Motherhood." In *Mothers in Law: Feminist Theory and the Legal Regulation of Motherhood*, edited by M.A. Fineman and I. Karpin. New York: Columbia University Press.

–. 1995b. "Race, Gender and the Value of Mothers' Work." *Social Politics* 2 (2): 195-207.

Roche, Maurice. 1992. *Rethinking Citizenship: Welfare, Ideology and Change in Modern Society*. Cambridge, UK: Polity Press.

Romanow, Roy J. 2002. *Shape the Future of Health Care: Interim Report*. Ottawa: Commission on the Future of Health Care in Canada.

Ross, David, Katherine Scott, and Mark A. Kelly. 1996. "Overview: Children in Canada in the 1990s." In *Growing Up in Canada: National Longitudinal Survey of Children and Youth*. Ottawa: Human Resources Development Canada/Statistics Canada.

Saharso, Sawitri. 2000. "Female Autonomy and Cultural Imperative: Two Hearts Beating Together." In *Citizenship in Diverse Societies*, edited by W. Kymlicka and W. Norman. Oxford, UK: Oxford University Press.

Sainsbury, Diane. 1996. *Gender, Equality, and Welfare States*. Cambridge: Cambridge University Press.

–, ed. 1994. *Gendering Welfare States*. London: Sage.

Sanchez, Laura, and Elizabeth Thomson. 1997. "Becoming Mothers and Fathers: Parenthood, Gender and the Division of Labor." *Gender and Society* 11 (6): 747-72.

Sandel, Michael J. 1984. "The Procedural Republic and the Unencumbered Self." *Political Theory* 12 (1): 81-96.

Sanderson, Susan, and Vetta L. Sanders Thompson. 2002. "Factors Associated with Perceived Paternal Involvement in Childrearing." *Sex Roles* 46 (3/4): 99-11.

Schabas, William A. 2000. "Freedom from Want: How Can We Make Indivisibility More than a Mere Slogan?" *Constitutional Law* 11 (2): 189-212.

Selbourne, David. 1994. *The Principle of Duty: An Essay on the Foundations of the Civic Order*. London: Sinclair Stevenson.

Shachar, Ayelet. 2000. "Should Church and State Be Joined at the Altar? Women's Rights and the Multicultural Dilemma." In *Citizenship in Diverse Societies*, edited by W. Kymlicka and W. Norman. Oxford, UK: Oxford University Press.

Shafir, Gershon. 1998. "Introduction: The Evolving Tradition of Citizenship." In *The Citizenship Debates*, edited by G. Shafir. Minneapolis: University of Minnesota Press.

Shaver, Sheila. 2002. "Australian Welfare Reform: From Citizenship to Supervision." *Social Policy and Administration* 36 (4): 331-45.

Sheridan, Mike, Deborah Sunter, and Brent Diverty. 1996. "The Changing Workweek: Trends in Weekly Hours of Work in Canada, 1976-1995." *Labour Force* 52 (6): C2-C31.

Siim, Birte. 1998. "Vocabularies of Citizenship and Gender: Denmark." *Critical Social Policy* 18 (3): 375-96.

Silver, Cynthia. 2000. "Being There: The Time Dual-Earner Couples Spend with Their Children." *Canadian Social Trends* (summer): 26-29.

Silverstein, Louise B., Carl F. Auerbach, Loretta Grieco, and Faith Dunkel. 1999. "Do Promise Keepers Dream of Feminist Sheep?" *Sex Roles* 40 (9/10): 665-88.

Slaughter, M.M. 1995. "The Legal Construction of 'Mother.'" In *Mothers in Law: Feminist Theory and the Legal Regulation of Motherhood,* edited by M.A. Fineman and I. Karpin. New York: Columbia University Press.

Smith, Beverley. 1997. "Complaint to Ms. Mongella, Deputy Director, Division for the Advancement of Women, United Nations Commission on the Status of Women." Copies of the complaint can be requested from <bevgsmith@ telusplanet.net>.

Statistics Canada. 1998. "1996 Census: Labour Force Activity, Occupation and Industry, Place of Work, Mode of Transportation to Work, Unpaid Work." *The Daily,* March 17. Available from http://www.statcan.ca/Daily/English/ 980317/d980317.htm.

–. 1999a. "Work Absence Rates, 1987 to 1998." Ottawa: Statistics Canada, Labour and Household Surveys Analysis Division. Catalogue no. 71-535-MPB, no. 10.

–. 1999b. "Employment Insurance Support to Families with Newborns." *The Daily,* October 25. Available from http://www.statcan.ca/Daily/English/991025/ d991025b.htm.

–. 1999c. "General Social Survey: Time Use." *The Daily,* 9 November 1999. Available from http://www.statcan.ca/Daily/English/991109/d991109a.htm.

–. 2000. "Women in Canada 2000: A Gender-Based Statistical Report." Ottawa: Statistics Canada, Housing, Family and Social Statistics Division.

Stewart, Angus. 2000. "Social Inclusion: An Introduction." In *Social Inclusion: Possibilities and Tensions,* edited by P. Askonas and A. Stewart. London: Macmillan.

Taylor, Charles. 1992. "Atomism." In *Communitarianism and Individualism,* edited by S. Avineri and A. De-Shalt. Oxford, UK: Oxford University Press.

–. 1994. "The Politics of Recognition." In *Multiculturalism,* edited by A. Gutman. Princeton, NJ: Princeton University Press.

Taylor-Goodby, Peter. 1991. *Social Change, Social Welfare and Social Science.* Toronto: University of Toronto Press.

Teghtsoonian, Katherine. 1997. "Who Pays for Caring for Children? Public Policy and the Devaluation of Women's Work." In *Challenging the Public/Private Divide: Feminism, Law, and Public Policy,* edited by S. Boyd. Toronto: University of Toronto Press.

Tougas, Jocelyne. 2002. "Reforming Quebec's Early Childhood Care and Education: The First Five Years." Toronto: Childcare Resource and Research Unit. Available from http://www.childcarecanada.org/pubs/op17/op17ENG.pdf.

Tronto, Joan C. 1993. *Moral Boundaries: A Political Argument for an Ethic of Care.* New York: Routledge.

Ursel, Jane. 1992. *Private Lives, Public Policy: 100 Years of State Intervention in the Family.* Toronto: Women's Press.

Walker, Alexis J., and Lori A. McGraw. 2000. "Who Is Responsible for Responsible Fathering?" *Journal of Marriage and the Family* 62: 563-69.

Walzer, Michael. 1991. "The Idea of Civil Society." *Dissent* 38 (spring): 293-304.

White, Deena. 2003. "Social Policy and Solidarity, Orphans and the New Model of Social Cohesion." *Canadian Journal of Sociology* 28 (1): 51-76.

White, Stuart. 2000. "Review Article: Social Rights and the Social Contract – Political Theory and the New Welfare Politics." *British Journal of Political Science* 30: 507-32.

–. 2003. *The Civic Minimum: On the Rights and Obligations of Economic Citizenship.* Oxford, UK: Oxford University Press.

Williams, Fiona. 1995. "Race/Ethnicity, Gender, and Class in Welfare States: A Framework for Comparative Analysis." *Social Politics* 2 (1): 127-59.

Workman, Thom. 1996. *Banking on Deception: The Discourse of Fiscal Crisis.* Halifax: Fernwood Publishing.

Zvonkovic, Anisa M., Kathleen M. Greaves, Cynthia J. Schmiege, and Leslie D. Hall. 1996. "The Marital Construction of Gender through Work and Family Decisions: A Qualitative Analysis." *Journal of Marriage and the Family* 58 (2): 91-100.

Index

31-32; state and citizenry care, 158-
59; entitlements vs, 2, 4, 13, 37, 48,
79-80, 124-25, 129, 145, 185; and
third way, 50-53; for welfare benefits,
85. *See also* social obligations
Oldfield, Adrian: on civic republicanism, 62-63, 63-64
Olson, Kevin: on choice and caregiving, 93, 155, 156, 157-58; on
paternalism, 138; rejects radical
daddy leave, 157
Ontario: child care in, 151; employment standards in, 134, 147, 158;
social assistance reductions in, 87;
wartime child care in, 76
Organization for Economic Cooperation and Development (OECD): on
fertility and female labour force
participation, 168; taxation in
OECD countries, 59; on young
households, 165
original position: 20, 25, 26, 29, 30,
33, 34-35, 65, 69, 70, 74
Orloff, Ann Shola, 102; on commodification, 78; on autonomous
households, 111
overtime work. *See under* paid work

paid work: choice not to engage in,
125; compatibility with unpaid
care, 184, 185; compatibility with
unpaid work, 187; domestic care
labour vs, 160-61; flexibility in
hours of, 149-50; high-tech sector,
134; hours of, 131, 133, 135, 154,
172; in information sector, 44; just-
in-time, 149-50; low-wage, 180;
overtime, 134, 146-47, 147-48, 149,
156, 173; part-time, 149-50; and
polarization of earnings, 173; reductions in hours of (*see* paid worktime
reductions); as requirement for
social assistance, 50; responsibility
to, 47; rest days from, 147; search
for, and receipt of social benefits,
79; in service sector, 53, 109, 133;
shortage of, 173; by single mothers,
125; and social citizenship, 75; as

social duty, 185; and social inclusion, 13, 123; time-banking system,
147. *See also* employment
paid workers: core, 133-34, 134, 135,
150; ideal, 134, 135, 138, 154, 161;
low-productivity, 165; part-time,
99, 139, 140, 148, 173; and retirement populations, 165; self-
employed, 140. *See also* labour
force; part-time workers
paid worktime, 132-33, 148; polarization in, 133-34; redistribution of,
174, 175, 177-78; weeks, 132-33,
146-47, 148, 150, 156, 172
paid worktime reductions, 146-50;
176-78; in Canada, 177; in Germany,
176-77
parental leave benefits, 57, 92, 103-4,
130, 165, 187; in Canada, 131-32;
under care*fair*, 143; changes under
care*fair*, 139-40; as citizenship
entitlement, 165; duration of, 139;
education and, 157; eligibility for,
139, 140; for fathers, 142-44, 156,
157; flat-rate, 123, 139, 140; incomes
and, 141; and low-income cut-off,
141; and moral hazard, 130-32,
138; and pension eligibility, 139-40,
145-46; and previous earnings,
140-41, 142, 143; in Spain, 175; in
Sweden, 172; symbolic coding of,
144-45; value of, 139, 140-42, 143;
and wage moderation strategies,
177-78; women as recipients, 90.
See also maternity leave benefits
parenting: deficit, 57, 92; and gender
division of labour, 131; as honour-
able vocation, 57-58; value of work,
81
parents: care as form of civic labour,
81-82; child care subsidies for low-
income, 101; and development of
moral norms, 72; divorced, 139;
lesbian, 139; low-income, 101; state
power over, 59-60; stay-at-home,
99; stress of, 186; work at home,
57. *See also* family/families; fathers;
mothers; single parents

172, 174, 175-77; and trends in
Scandinavia, 168-69, 172, 175-76;
and trends in US, 170, 174; and
work-family balance, 185. *See also*
paid worktime
Tocqueville, Alexis de, 1-2, 21, 62, 63
training-fare, 43
trampoline metaphor of citizenship,
4, 179
transfer dependency, 41-42, 43-44,
48, 49, 51, 53, 86-87
Tronto, Joan C., 68, 72, 79

unemployment, 165, 174, 185;
anticipated vs unanticipated, 42;
benefits, 51, 52; and leave benefits,
176; rates, 87; state responsibility
for, 31; structural, 86, 180; and
teeter-totter metaphor, 181; as
voluntary, 86; and workfare, 82;
and worktime redistribution, 175.
See also joblessness
unemployment insurance, 41-42,
87, 93
unencumbered self, 33-34, 36, 74, 76
United States: Cost, Quality and
Child Outcomes (CQO) study, 167;
earnings in, 170; infants in parental
care, 172; paid hours in, 170; time
trends in, 170, 174
universal breadwinner model of
citizenship, 98, 101, 104
universal caregiver model of citizenship, 10, 84-85, 92, 138, 155, 156,
157

values, 33, 34; family, 59
veil of ignorance, 20, 29, 33, 35
victim-blaming, 49
voluntary sector, 4

Walzer, Michael, 54, 64; on civil
society, 182
Weber, Max: definition of state, 159
welfare: and African American
mothers, 110; benefits for children,
43; and class-based analyses, 29-30;
at community level, 53;

contractualism, 2; contributions
made within private sphere, 29-30,
84; cost vs effect on poor, 48; cross-
cultural differences, 158; dependence upon, 110 (*see also* transfer
dependency); diamond, 3, 13; and
duty discourses, 17; and duty to
work, 48; employment obligations
and, 85; as entitlement, 48; equality
and, 50; and families, 58-59; and
family values, 59; generosity of, 43;
and human capital, 11; and income
level, 11; inequalities in systems,
130; and institutionalization of
incentives, 42; and market participation, 11, 183; market vs, 158;
market-income equivalencies, 43;
passivity of policy, 50; paternalism
in, 156; permissive vs authoritative
programs, 47; postwar services, 2, 3;
and private sphere, 183; provision
by state, 3; provision by women in
home, 76; as reciprocal contract,
48. 50; and safety net metaphor,
179; and single mothers, 59; and
social conservatives, 58; and social
investment state, 78, 179; social
liberal focus on, 32; and social
obligations, 48; as social right, 80;
state restructuring and, 45; state- vs
market-based, 47; and subsidized
housing, 43; tax base for, 31; tax
rates for people leaving, 43; taxation
to fund, 59; and teeter-totter
metaphor, 181-82; and third way,
52-53; and traditional family, 61;
and "training-fare," 43-44; and
trampoline metaphor, 4, 179; trap,
42-43; unpaid, in domestic sphere,
83-84; and voluntary associations,
53; and wage system, 31; wall, 6;
work requirements for, 50; and
workfare, 43-44. *See also* social
assistance
welfare contractualism: and care*fair*,
129, 187; feminism and, 78; and
justice, 79; Mead's vision of, 48-49;
and reciprocity, 160; and social